Discord

EPIDEMICS

GREAT DISASTERS

EPIDEMICS

Other books in the Great Disasters series:

GREAT DISASTERS

EPIDEMICS

Lisa Yount, *Book Editor*

Daniel Leone, *President*
Bonnie Szumski, *Publisher*
Scott Barbour, *Managing Editor*

GREENHAVEN
PRESS®

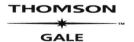

THOMSON
—✳—
GALE
™

San Diego • Detroit • New York • San Francisco • Cleveland
New Haven, Conn. • Waterville, Maine • London • Munich

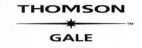

LIBRARY OF CONGRESS CATALOGING-IN-PUBLICATION DATA

Epidemics / Lisa Yount, book editor.
    p. cm. — (Great disasters)
    Includes bibliographical references and index.
    ISBN 0-7377-1442-5 (pbk. : alk. paper) — ISBN 0-7377-1441-7 (lib. : alk. paper)
        1. Epidemics—Popular works. 2. Epidemiology—Popular works. I. Yount, Lisa.
    II. Series.
    RA653.E655 2003
    614.4—dc21   2003040759

Printed in the United States of America

CONTENTS

FOREWORD

Humans have an ambivalent relationship with their home planet, nurtured on the one hand by Earth's bounty but devastated on the other hand by its catastrophic natural disasters. While these events are the results of the natural processes of Earth, their consequences for humans frequently include the disastrous destruction of lives and property. For example, when the volcanic island of Krakatau exploded in 1883, the eruption generated vast seismic sea waves called tsunamis that killed about thirty-six thousand people in Indonesia. In a single twenty-four-hour period in the United States in 1974, at least 148 tornadoes carved paths of death and destruction across thirteen states. In 1976, an earthquake completely destroyed the industrial city of Tangshan, China, killing more than 250,000 residents.

Some natural disasters have gone beyond relatively localized destruction to completely alter the course of human history. Archaeological evidence suggests that one of the greatest natural disasters in world history happened in A.D. 535, when an Indonesian "supervolcano" exploded near the same site where Krakatau arose later. The dust and debris from this gigantic eruption blocked the light and heat of the sun for eighteen months, radically altering weather patterns around the world and causing crop failure in Asia and the Middle East. Rodent populations increased with the weather changes, causing an epidemic of bubonic plague that decimated entire populations in Africa and Europe. The most powerful volcanic eruption in recorded human history also happened in Indonesia. When the volcano Tambora erupted in 1815, it ejected an estimated 1.7 million tons of debris in an explosion that was heard more than a thousand miles away and that continued to rumble for three months. Atmospheric dust from the eruption blocked much of the sun's heat, producing what was called "the year without summer" and creating worldwide climatic havoc, starvation, and disease.

As these examples illustrate, natural disasters can have as much impact on human societies as the bloodiest wars and most chaotic political revolutions. Therefore, they are as worthy of study as the

major events of world history. As with the study of social and
political events, the exploration of natural disasters can illuminate
the causes of these catastrophes and target the lessons learned
about how to mitigate and prevent the loss of life when disaster
strikes again. By examining these events and the forces behind
them, the Greenhaven Press Great Disasters series is designed to
help students better understand such cataclysmic events. Each anthology in the series focuses on a specific type of natural disaster or a particular disastrous event in history. An introductory essay provides a general overview of the subject of the anthology,
placing natural disasters in historical and scientific context. The
essays that follow, written by specialists in the field, researchers,
journalists, witnesses, and scientists, explore the science and nature of natural disasters, describing particular disasters in detail
and discussing related issues, such as predicting, averting, or managing disasters. To aid the reader in choosing appropriate material, each essay is preceded by a concise summary of its content
and biographical information about its author.

In addition, each volume contains extensive material to help
the student researcher. An annotated table of contents and a
comprehensive index help readers quickly locate particular subjects of interest. To guide students in further research, each volume features an extensive bibliography including books, period-
icals, and related Internet websites. Finally, appendixes provide
glossaries of terms, tables of measurements, chronological charts
of major disasters, and related materials. With its many useful features, the Greenhaven Press Great Disasters series offers students
a fascinating and awe-inspiring look at the deadly power of
Earth's natural forces and their catastrophic impact on humans.

INTRODUCTION

The Book of Revelation, the last book of the Bible's New Testament, pictures four terrible horsemen bringing disaster to humankind. The last horseman, on his "pale horse," is often held to represent plague, or pestilence—in other words, epidemic diseases. In placing epidemics in the fearsome company of such mighty forces as war and famine (the second and third horsemen), the writer of that ancient book showed a keen, though probably intuitive, sense of history. Many modern historians agree that epidemics have not only brought sickness and death to millions but have produced effects, subtle or striking, on events far removed in time or space from the waves of illness themselves.

"Disease has to be counted as one of the wild cards of history, an unforeseen factor that can, in a matter of days or weeks, undo the deterministic sure thing or humble the conquering momentum," writes William H. McNeill, a University of Chicago emeritus professor and winner of the National Book Award and the Erasmus Award. "Bacteria and viruses may . . . redirect vast impersonal forces in human societies, and they can also become forces in their own right."

Disease historians such as Arno Karlen, a psychoanalyst who has written such books as *Man and Microbes* and *Biography of a Germ,* believe that epidemics and human history in fact, evolved together. Infectious diseases—those caused by microorganisms and other small parasites—have surely always existed in humans, as they do in animals, but epidemics could occur only after large numbers of people began to live close together; thus, epidemics began to occur when cities (and, at about the same time, written history) developed. In an epidemic, disease-causing microorganisms spread quickly and strike many people in the same area at about the same time. Living conditions in cities, past and present, allow easy spread of microbes through direct contact, contaminated food and water, and insect pests such as mosquitoes and fleas. The epidemic ends only when virtually everyone in an area has either died or become immune, meaning able to resist the attacks of that type of microorganism.

Examples of epidemics that altered history date back to ancient times. For instance, McNeill mentions the fact that an epidemic of unknown nature among the soldiers of Sennacherib, king of Assyria, was a major reason why Sennacherib abandoned his seige of Jerusalem, capital of the tiny kingdom of Judah, in 701 B.C. The epidemic thus both preserved the kingdom and strengthened its people's belief in a single God, since they saw the plague as an act of God's protection. McNeill believes that if the Assyrians had conquered Jerusalem, its inhabitants probably would have been killed or scattered and their civilization destroyed. "If so, Judaism would have disappeared from the face of the earth and the two daughter religions of Christianity and Islam could not possibly have come into existence. In short, our world would be profoundly different in ways we cannot really imagine."

Epidemics have contributed to destroying civilizations as well as saving them. Karlen cites the Plague of Athens, an epidemic that struck that ancient Greek city-state at the height of its power, during the "golden age" of Pericles and Socrates, in 430 B.C. This plague, also of an unknown type, not only killed a third of Athens's citizens but, Karlen says, indirectly led to the city's losing the Peloponnesian War against rival Sparta and, ultimately, its collapse. "With its great naval power, Athens should have been able to outlast Sparta," Karlen writes. "Without the plague, it might have. . . . [After losing the war] Athens would never fully regain its political or cultural glory."

Other epidemics produced far more widespread effects. Disease historians including Canadian writer Andrew Nikiforuk and Scripps Research Institute member Michael B.A. Oldstein maintain that the native civilizations of the Americas succumbed chiefly to smallpox, not to the might of European armies. This virus-caused illness had spread death and disfigurement through Europe and Asia since ancient times, so by the time Spanish conquistador Hernán Cortés and his handful of soldiers arrived in Tenochtitlán in 1521, most Europeans had been exposed to the disease in childhood, and survivors were immune. The Aztecs and other natives, on the other hand, had never encountered the virus and therefore had absolutely no resistance to it. When the Europeans accidentally introduced the disease, the native Americans died by the millions. Furthermore, seeing the Europeans untouched by the epidemic helped to convince the natives that the invaders had superhuman powers—a belief that worked to the advantage of the conquerors.

A different epidemic disease, yellow fever, helped to shape the history of slavery. This illness, which is spread by mosquitoes, is common in Africa, and many Africans were resistant to it, just as Europeans were to smallpox. Some of the first Africans brought to the Americas as slaves carried the yellow fever virus in their blood, and when American mosquitoes bit them and then bit Europeans or Native Americans, who had been enslaved earlier in large numbers, they introduced the disease into populations as helpless before it as the natives had been before smallpox. In this case, though, their resistance brought the Africans increased slavery rather than victory because it added to their value as workers in the tropical climates where yellow fever-carrying mosquitoes flourished.

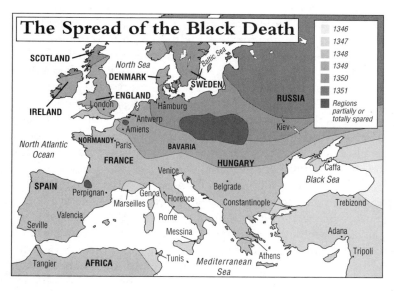

Epidemic diseases are thought to have been the hidden forces behind many specific historic events, great and small. For example, the French emperor Napoléon sent twenty-seven thousand soldiers to put down a slave rebellion in Haiti in 1802, but most of the soldiers succumbed instead to yellow fever. This epidemic not only preserved Haiti's newly won independence but convinced Napoléon that defending the much larger French territory in North America would be impractical. As a result, he sold that immense tract of land to the United States a year later for a bargain price, allowing the fledgling country to more than double in size and helping to guarantee its eventual rise to world power.

The nineteenth and early twentieth centuries brought a better understanding of causes of infectious diseases and how they spread, as well as the development of vaccines against major killers such as smallpox, yellow fever, and polio. These developments, as well as the discovery of antibiotics during the 1940s, led many people in developed countries to believe that, as then-Surgeon General William S. Stewart said in 1967, such countries could "close the book on epidemic diseases." Symbolizing such hopes, following an intensive vaccination campaign, the World Health Organization announced the eradication of natural smallpox worldwide during the late 1970s.

Even as the announcement was made, however, evidence began to grow that epidemics' effects on world history were far from over. Microbes that caused familiar diseases such as tuberculosis showed signs of resistance to drugs that had formerly slain them. Seemingly new and dramatically deadly infections such as Ebola fever appeared in obscure parts of the world freshly invaded by human settlement. Far more stealthy, but ultimately worst of all, was the disease that spread from its first reported occurrences in handfuls of homosexual men and users of injected drugs to become a worldwide plague affecting millions of people: AIDS. As the twenty-first century began, furthermore, fears grew that bioterrorists might deliberately start epidemics of smallpox, anthrax, or other fatal diseases.

Possible terrorist attacks are only one form in which epidemic disease may affect the world history of today and tomorrow. Chronic infectious diseases such as malaria sap the strength of the citizens of many developing countries, helping to keep those countries poor. Aided by rapid worldwide travel and trade, "emerging" infections such as West Nile fever and SARS (Sudden Acute Respiratory Syndrome) appear in spots far from their origin and could develop into major health threats. Most importantly, AIDS is destroying an entire generation in Africa and, probably, Asia and Eastern Europe as well. By mid-2002, 20 million people had died from this disease and 40 million were believed to be infected, and Peter Piot, executive director of the Joint United Nations Programme on HIV/AIDS (UNAIDS), said that the epidemic was still "in its early stages." He estimated that 70 million people would die of the disease during the next twenty years. AIDS, which preferentially strikes young adults in their most productive years, is wiping out police officers, teachers, and other essential jobholders throughout Africa, causing social and economic devastation of unimaginable proportions, and the same may shortly be true of India, China, and other Asian countries.

Have no doubt about it—the fourth horseman still rides.

The Science of Epidemics

The Evolution of Epidemics

By Arno Karlen

Microorganisms are the cause of infectious diseases, says psychoanalyst Arno Karlen, but epidemics, in which the same disease infects many people at the same time, arise because of certain human behaviors. Karlen explains that epidemics became possible only after the development of cities, in which large numbers of people crowded together and, often, ate poor diets and allowed human or animal excrement to foul their water and food. He describes the ways epidemic diseases have spread throughout history and how human actions have contributed to this process. Karlen's books about history and biomedical topics include Biography of a Germ, *the story of the microorganism that causes Lyme disease.*

From Babylon to Paris, the metropolis has evoked images of splendor and apocalypse. Thomas Wolfe, the prototypical small-town boy infatuated with big cities, called them "the places where we feel our lives will be gloriously fulfilled, our hungers fed." For variety and possibilities, they equal anything in nature. No tropical forest surpasses London or Paris in richness of life, no mountain is more stunning than Manhattan's skyline, no valley more inviting than the streets of Amsterdam. Cities promise new pleasures, risks, friends, lovers, fortunes. They are the electrical poetry of group life.

Cities, however, have also inspired a dark poetry of decay and misfortune. From Petronius [an ancient Roman writer] to [Charles] Dickens and [Emile] Zola, writers have seen the metropolis as a warren of corruption, poverty, violence, and disease. The very existence of cities seems to bring fear that the hubris of creating them will be punished by disaster and collapse. They evoke images of the swamp and the jungle. The feeling has some

Arno Karlen, *Man and Microbes: Disease and Plagues in History and Modern Times.* New York: G.P. Putnam's Sons, 1995. Copyright © 1995 by Quantum Research Associates, Inc. Reproduced by permission.

basis in reality. From their beginnings until the twentieth century, cities have been pestholes. In fact, only when towns became big cities did massive die-offs become a regular part of human life. The author of the Book of Revelation saw the lethal side of cities: "He that is in the field shall die with the sword; and he that is in the city, famine and pestilence shall devour him."

Why Epidemics Need Cities

When farmers and villagers began crowding into cities, this immunologically virgin mass offered a feast to germs lurking in domesticated animals, wastes, filth, and scavengers. Countless people were sickened and killed by previously unknown epidemics—smallpox, measles, mumps, influenza, scarlet fever, typhus, bubonic plague, syphilis, gonorrhea, and the common cold. Many of these diseases attacked with a savagery they rarely show today, demoralizing entire societies. If we are to see why new epidemics are again striking an increasingly urbanized world, we must understand why plagues and cities have always developed together.

For several million years, the main causes of human deaths were accidents and wounds. Permanent farms and villages made death by disease far more frequent. Then the population explosion of the Bronze Age, 6,000 years ago, took city dwellers beyond a crucial threshold. Urban masses became sufficiently large and dense to support zymotics, or crowd diseases, what in other species are called herd diseases. For the first time, infection became humanity's chief cause of death. Despite a few respites, this would remain true in the West until this century. Infections are still the main killers in many poor nations, and they recurrently threaten the rich ones.

The reason epidemics did not take hold until urban times is simply the conditions imposed by numbers. While nomads were not free of infection, their most common diseases were chronic, not acute. Deadly epidemics remained relatively limited and infrequent for the same reasons they had been so among hunter-gatherers. People did not live densely packed together, aiding transmission of germs from one person to another. Their settlements were sufficiently far apart, and travel was sufficiently limited, to keep outbreaks of diseases localized.

Furthermore, most bacterial and viral infections with epidemic potential leave survivors temporarily or permanently immune. When such diseases did jump from an animal source to nomads or villagers, they flashed through the population; soon most of the people in a community were either dead or immune. The microbes, having run out of susceptible hosts, died off. Only years or generations later could the germ attack successfully again, de-

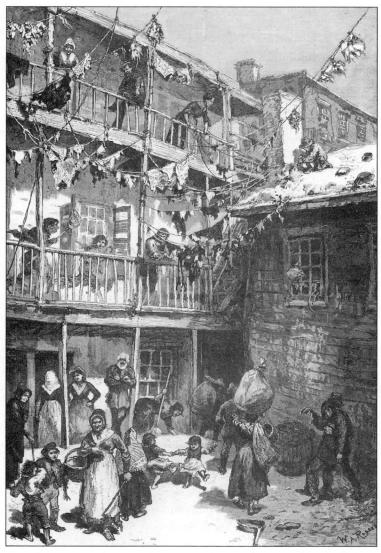

Crowded living conditions, such as in this 1879 tenement in New York City, aid the transmission of germs to many people, allowing epidemics to spread.

pending on a new crop of susceptibles and another accident of reintroduction. Writers often speak of crowd diseases with the metaphor of fire, and of human hosts as fuel. If there is too little fuel or if it is too thinly scattered, the blaze sputters out. The image, though simplistic, is basically accurate. In epidemiologists' terms, a zymotic persists only if the population is dense enough to keep transmitting the germs and big enough to keep producing new susceptibles. Herd diseases jump from animals to humans and thrive only if the people form a superherd. Once cities hold several thousand people, they can support most present-day crowd diseases. That first happened in the ancient Middle East. . . .

How Epidemics Spread

About half of all human infections are spread by microscopic droplets breathed, coughed, or sneezed into the air. Crowded, poorly ventilated ancient cities were Eden for such diseases, from measles and mumps to tuberculosis. The most common of all crowd diseases, the common cold—more accurately colds, similar conditions caused by a hundred or so related viruses—is airborne. Since they infect only humans and horses, these viruses doubtless are descended from some grandmother of all colds that made the leap from domesticated horses to people four or five thousand years ago.

Disease germs that spread by direct body contact became more common and severe. Skin diseases are common but usually mild among villagers in warm, moist climates; they are transmitted easily among playing children by the touch of perspiring skin. As settled populations grew, especially in temperate climates, fullbody clothing became customary year round; germs that infected the skin found their usual homes and means of transmission threatened. They took refuge in warm, moist parts of the body, where they could survive during longer intervals between skin contacts of hosts. That is, they settled in and around the mouth, genitals, and anus, awaiting sexual transmission. Thus they became diseases not of children but of adolescents and adults. In cities, the rise in each person's number of potential sex partners allowed gonorrhea and syphilis to become rampant. Prostitution, a regular trade at least several thousand years ago, created a new pool of people who were at once victims and sources of sexually transmitted diseases.

Deadly Water

Waterborne germs are transmitted by drinking and bathing and by tainted food, fingers, and household implements. Their usual ultimate source is human or animal feces, which Bronze Age cities produced in prodigious amounts. Fecally contaminated water can spread polio, cholera, viral hepatitis, whooping cough, diphtheria, typhoid, and paratyphoid fever. Most of these diseases adapted to urban people from their original homes in domestic animals and scavengers. Typhoid, for instance, is often fatal to humans, but rarely severe in rodents and birds, which are thought to be the original hosts.

Typhoid is one of many diseases caused by *Salmonella* bacteria; literally thousands of types of these bacteria live in warm-blooded species. Well into this century, *Salmonella* infections were a leading cause of fatal infant diarrhea. They still cause food poisoning in people of all ages, mostly through poultry and eggs, but sometimes through vegetables washed in infected water or touched by unwashed hands. Similarly, contaminated milk, meat, and vegetables can transmit diphtheria, brucellosis, tuberculosis, and other infections.

Another nasty waterborne germ is the *Shigella* bacterium. It has no known animal reservoir but primates; it probably adapted to man from monkeys that raided farmers' crops or that lived near people, as the temple monkeys of India still do. Shigellosis remains common in Africa, and it causes more intestinal infections in developed nations, including the United States, than was once supposed. It has also become a sexually transmitted disease, thanks to a variety of anal-erotic flippancies—a warning that a zoonosis, having found one means of human-to-human transmission, may find still others.

Crawling and Flying

Finally, infections are spread by vectors, creatures that carry them to other species, with or without being affected. Rodents, birds, and snails can carry pathogens to humans, but by far the most varied and numerous vectors are arthropods—organisms with jointed external skeletons such as insects and ticks. Early cities and their disrupted environs gave new homes to countless arthropods, such as beetles, bedbugs, mites, and mosquitoes. They invaded fields, gardens, houses, granaries, refuse heaps, animal pens, even clothes, bedding, and dust. Among the arbo (short for "arthropod-borne") infections that adapted to humans are malignant tertian malaria, yellow fever, dengue, sleeping sickness, typhus, typhus's rickettsial relatives, and the recently arrived Lyme disease.

Some of those germs adapted exclusively to people; others remained able to infect their original hosts and vectors as well. Being at home in two or more species gives a germ obvious advantages. It is more likely to survive the temporary or prolonged absence of one type of host; and a mobile host or vector, such as a bird or mosquito, can extend the germ's geographic range and its number of victims. Such adaptability is a double lease on life in times of ecological disruption. And the growth of early cities and their surrounding fields created disruptions on a monumental scale.

The Mystery of Disease

When Bronze Age cities were inviting so many new germs and means of transmissions, some social customs may have retarded the spread of infections slightly. The Hebrews expelled individuals with severe skin diseases and, like Hindus and Muslims, required frequent ritual washing with water or sand. Historians have guessed that some dietary laws, such as the Hebrew ban on pork and shellfish, rose from knowledge that these foods could pass on diseases such as trichinosis and hepatitis. It seems more likely that these practices reflected ideas of ritual purity or magical taboo; the idea of infection in its modern sense was unknown.

Even if Bronze Age people had known why new diseases were striking them, that knowledge probably wouldn't have helped much. They still would have had no cures and few preventives. Population pressure still would have forced them to disrupt their ecosystems by land clearance for farming and herding, and to change their daily lives with new technology, trade, and living conditions. Anyway, they did not know where new diseases came from; they could explain them only as divine punishment, and pray in vain for relief.

From about 4000 B.C. to A.D. 400, the onslaught of new diseases continued, as people were exposed to germs they had met rarely during the millions of years when their immune systems had evolved. Fortunately, these did not all appear at once, in part because each has its own population threshold. But once those thresholds were breached, epidemics swept through cities and then spilled into surrounding towns and villages. The villagers had been exposed to fewer germs as they grew up, so their immune defenses were, in the metaphor of epidemiologists, naive. Therefore they may have been hit even harder than city dwellers. . . .

It is chilling to think that . . . [the] plague [of Athens in 430 B.C.] was probably no worse than many other epidemics of the Bronze and Iron ages. But more important for history than its virulence was its origin. According to Thucydides, it came by ship from Africa. If so, this is the first recorded instance of the spread of a crowd disease from one of the world's major centers of infection to another.

War, Trade, and Travel

Long before the golden age of Athens, foci [centers] of infections had developed in Mediterranean Europe, Egypt, Mesopotamia, India, and China. Each area, with its own climate, ecosystem, and germs, had a distinctive set of infections, to which people adapted with a distinctive complex of immune defenses. By the time of the plague of Athens, the foci of Egypt and Mesopotamia had probably fused and come into contact with that of India. India's may have already brushed China's. But only with Thucydides' account do we have a documented episode in the emergence of a band of common infections across Eurasia and North Africa. For pathogens, these foci were merging and becoming one. The reasons were war and travel.

There are other ancient mentions of plagues, and those records of devastation and despair hold signs that a common pool of zymotics was emerging across the urbanized Old World. In the fourteenth century B.C., a Hittite priest bemoaned a plague that had been killing his people since their contact with Egyptian prisoners of war twenty years earlier. He wrote that "men have been dying in my father's days, in my brother's days, and in mine. . . . The agony in my heart and the anguish in my soul I cannot endure any more." Fields went unplowed and bread unbaked, because farmers and grinding women were dead. Sheepfolds and cow pens were empty; the shepherds and cowherds had perished. The priest prayed in vain to a river god he thought had sent the plague to punish the Hittites for failing to keep a wartime pledge to the deity. His lament, still poignant across 3,400 years, tells us that the Hittite plague, like the plague of Athens, was the poisoned fruit of military power.

More and more epidemics were spreading across the world by

travel, trade, and war. There were more people, bigger armies, better transport. By 6,000 years ago, the Egyptians had boats that could carry cargo and troops; 500 years later, so did the Mesopotamians. Knossos, in Bronze Age Crete, was the hub of a trade network connecting Europe and the Near East. By Roman times, cargo ships weighing more than a thousand tons traded between Italy and India. People carried diseases by ship and camel caravan, across seas and mountains and deserts; with them went stowaway pests, the germs of ship rats, and livestock parasites. By late Roman days, every major urban society in the Old World probably had passed zymotics to several others, causing the sort of devastation that had struck the Hittites and Athenians.

Diseases kept spreading because humans responded to their population explosion just as other social species do. They fought for more resources, sought new territories, tested neighbors' boundaries. Some migrated westward from India across Europe, carrying the Indo-European languages. In the Middle and Near East, the clash of growing populations brought the rise and fall of Sumerians, Akkadians, Babylonians, Kassites, Hittites, Egyptians, Assyrians, Chaldeans, and Persians. Later, tribes that would be called Germanic and central European pushed at the boundaries of the Roman empire and finally broke through. Everywhere, venturesome hordes and armies visited new diseases on lands they occupied, and tribal masses fell victim to infections of the cities they conquered. To microbes, both sides in these struggles were just fresh meat.

The Weakeners

As fearsome as new epidemics were in the Bronze and Iron ages, less dramatic endemics [diseases constantly present in a region] probably caused just as much damage. Malaria and schistosomiasis flourished in the farms and villages that now covered more and more of the earth to feed cities' appetites. This was especially true where warm climates combined with irrigation to create something like the ideal environment of many parasites, that of the rain forest.

The signs of these ancient infections are ubiquitous. The mud-brick walls of ancient Mesopotamian cities contain shells of the *Bulinus* snail, which harbors the schistosome. Greece and Rome suffered badly from malaria; Hippocrates and Galen described three of its four varieties with perfect clinical clarity. Then, as today, endemic malaria and schistosomiasis created a debilitated peasantry, many of them too sick to work, victimized by other epidemics, and destined to early death. By draining people's vigor, such endemics stole the cities' lifeblood.

As cities enhanced old diseases and fostered new ones, births could not keep up with deaths. To replace the casualties of crowd diseases and maintain their populations, cities needed a constant inflow of migrants from the countryside. There were always willing farmers and villagers; when diseases took their rural toll, many of the men who survived fled hopefully to the economic promise of cities. One sees a result of this today in many Third World countries, where only the old, the sick, women, and children remain to work the land. Many ancient empires must have fallen because the peasants were sickly, their ranks thinned by migration to cities harrowed by epidemics.

Cities Survived

It is a testimony to human vigor and adaptability that city life flourished despite plagues, famines, wars, and migrations. The assault by new crowd diseases was fierce and unrelenting. A human population usually needs at least a century or so to stabilize in response to an unfamiliar infection. Through the Bronze and Iron ages, people had to endure that struggle again and again, often with only brief respites. No sooner did they reach relative tolerance of a new epidemic than another arrived, caught from an animal source or a foreign focus of infection.

Cities not only survived, they grew in size and number. Catastrophic epidemics were followed by resurging populations and renewed urban growth. There are economic and biological explanations, based on models of population dynamics and resource exploitation; some of these are plausible and probably partly true. I suggest, however, that the primary force driving urban growth was something in the human temperament—a combination of curiosity, inventiveness, and hunger for stimulation.

Laboratory rats and monkeys will exhaust or even kill themselves if they are allowed to keep artificially stimulating themselves, whether with sweets, energizing drugs, or electrical jolts to the brain. We, too, are fools for stimulation. The variety and excitement of city life are super stimuli. Humans, with much greater capacities for excitement and boredom than other creatures, have a hard time resisting those stimuli. Like rats or rhesus monkeys that will binge on sugar, cocaine, or brain shocks despite the noxious results, people risk discomfort or even death to be in environments full of challenge and adventure. Evolution has encouraged us to do so by sharpening and prolonging the curiosity and playfulness that in most species end with childhood.

But the human immune system is not infinitely adaptable. The biological price of urbanization, trade, travel, and war was increased saturation with infections across much of the Old World. Technology had allowed diseases to multiply and travel, but it could not yet offer ways to combat them. Finally the human burden of disease became so great that only the end of urban life could relieve it. Humanity experienced a population crash, of a kind some scientists fear may once again lie in our future.

The Threat of Epidemics Today

By Hilary French

Many people think that antibiotics and other medical advances have made epidemics a thing of the past, at least in developed countries. However, Hilary French, an environmental protection expert, claims that this is far from true. She explains how rapid worldwide travel and trade, coupled with environmental destruction and growing settlements in areas where few or no humans have previously lived, encourage disease-causing microorganisms to spread far from their place of origin. As a result, she says, an epidemic anywhere in the world becomes the concern of everyone. French is a staff member of the Worldwatch Institute, a nonprofit research organization specializing in international environmental and development issues. Her writings include Vanishing Borders: Protecting the Planet in the Age of Globalization.

For most of history, natural boundaries such as mountains, deserts, and ocean currents have served to isolate ecosystems and many of the species they contain. However, these physical barricades are now becoming permeable as people and organisms spread around the globe, leading to ecological disruptions with damaging and unpredictable consequences.

Ecological integration has accelerated dramatically in recent decades, as trade and travel have skyrocketed. More than 5,000,000,000 tons of goods are being shipped across the world's oceans and other waterways annually. International air travel is also soaring. More people are flying greater distances than ever before, with 2,000,000 crossing an international border every day. Since 1950, the number of passenger-miles flown has increased at an average of nine percent.

The rapid growth in the movement of human beings and

Hilary French, "Travel and Trade: Hidden Threats," *USA Today*, vol. 129, March 2001, p. 56. Copyright © 2001 by Society for the Advancement of Education. Reproduced by permission.

their goods and services around the world has provided convenient transportation for thousands of other species of plants and animals that are taking root on foreign shores. This explosion in the movement of species and microbes across international borders poses a major threat to both the planet's biological diversity and the health of its human inhabitants. . . .

Microbes Across Borders

In the first centuries of the Roman Empire, growing commerce between Mediterranean civilizations and Asia precipitated the great plague of 165 A.D. Believed to have been smallpox, this epidemic claimed the lives of a quarter of the population of the Roman Empire. In the 14th century, bubonic plague swept through Europe—the Black Death. This epidemic, which caused the deaths of a third of Europe's population, was introduced into China as the Mongol empire expanded across central Asia, and from there spread by caravan routes to the Crimea and the Mediterranean. Today, the process of globalization is dramatically accelerating the pace at which microbes travel the globe. As the late AIDS researcher Jonathan Mann of Harvard University explained, "The world has rapidly become much more vulnerable to the eruption and . . . to the widespread and even global spread of both new and old infectious diseases. This new and heightened vulnerability isn't mysterious. The dramatic increase in worldwide movement of people, goods, and ideas is the driving force behind the globalization of disease." Only by looking out for the health of people everywhere is it possible to promote healthy societies anywhere.

The rapid growth in international air travel is a particularly potent force for global disease dissemination, as air travel makes it possible for people to reach the other side of the world far quicker than the incubation period for many ailments. At the same time, adventure tourism and other pursuits are drawing people to more-remote locations, increasing the chance that microbes will be introduced to vulnerable populations.

"Sick" Environments Produce Sick People

Environmental degradation is another powerful contributor to many of today's most pressing global health threats. The World Health Organization (WHO) estimates that nearly a quarter of the global burden of disease and injury is related to environmental disruption and decline. For certain diseases, the environmental contribution is far greater. About 90% of diarrheal diseases such as cholera, which kill 3,000,000 people a year, result from contaminated water. Moreover, 90% of the 1,500,000–2,700,000 deaths caused by malaria annually are linked with underlying environmental disruptions such as the colonization of rainforests and the construction of large open-water irrigation schemes, both of which increase human exposure to disease-carrying mosquitoes. A 1998 analysis by Cornell University ecologist David Pimentel and his colleagues reached an even starker

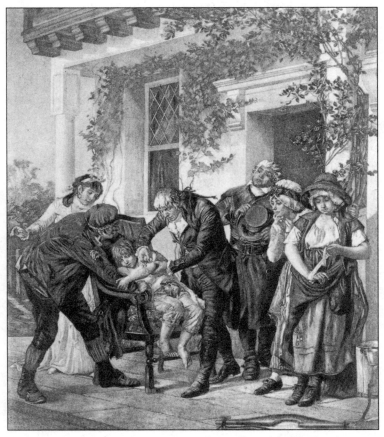

This picture portrays the first vaccination for smallpox, by Dr. Edward Jenner. Despite medical advances such as vaccination, epidemics still can spread quickly, due to increasing worldwide travel and trade.

conclusion—that around 40% of all deaths worldwide are attributable to environmental decline.

When globalization and environmental decline join forces, the health implications can be staggering. The power of this combination is demonstrated by the tragic history of the AIDS pandemic. As of 1999, the HIV virus had infected 50,000,000 people worldwide, killing more than 16,000,000. In particularly hard-hit countries in Africa, as much as a quarter of the population harbors the virus.

The epidemic initially came to light at roughly the same time in the early 1980s in Africa, the Caribbean, and North America. The question of where the virus had originated was politically charged, with WHO skirting the issue for many years by maintaining that the virus had emerged simultaneously on at least three continents. "Few scientists accepted that position, recognizing it for what it was—a political compromise," notes author Laurie Garrett in *The Coming Plague*. "If humanity hoped to prevent its next great plague, it was vital to understand the origins of this one." In the last few years, scientists have made important strides toward getting to the bottom of this controversial question.

It is now widely believed that HIV was originally harbored in chimpanzees inhabiting the West African rainforest, crossing over into human populations as early as the 1940s. Although exactly how this occurred will never be known, scientists speculate that it resulted from hunters cutting themselves while harvesting their kill, or perhaps through the direct consumption of raw meat. The epidemic thus may have had its origins in intermingling between humans and chimpanzees as a result of human incursion into previously remote forests. According to a theory put forth by Jaap Goudsmit of the University of Amsterdam, the decline in chimpanzee populations resulting from the human invasion might have created a biological imperative for the simian immunodeficiency viruses to seek out new hosts—humans.

Scientists believe that saving Africa's imperiled chimpanzees may be crucial for discovering a way to stave off the deadly HIV infection in humans, as the animals are immune from HIV's most lethal effects. Africa's primates are under siege, though, with many on the verge of extinction. One major threat is the thriving "bushmeat" trade. As logging roads penetrate remote forests, loggers and hunters snare chimpanzees, gorillas, monkeys, bush pigs, snakes, and other prey. They either eat the meat themselves or transport it to West African cities, where bushmeat is considered a delicacy. "These chimps are information we need," maintains Beatrice Hahn of the University of Alabama, who led a team in 1999 that confirmed the link between AIDS and chimps. "Killing them for the pot is like burning a library full of books you haven't read yet," she argues.

Worldwide Highways to Disaster

Another major outstanding question related to the origins of the AIDS epidemic is how HIV, once it was transferred from chimps to humans, made the leap from being an isolated condition confined to Africa's remote hinterlands to its current status as a global pandemic. Although many links in this chain are unknown, a range of phenomena are thought to have contributed, including warfare near the region where the virus is believed to have first emerged; the paving of the TransAfrica highway, which provided an easy route for carrying HIV across the continent; population growth and urbanization; and, ultimately, burgeoning international travel and migration.

As the movement of people into remote parts of West Africa's forests continues to pick up speed thanks to logging and hunting, scientists warn that other dangerous viruses may make the jump from primates to people. An even broader issue is at stake as well. "AIDS is trying to teach us a lesson," Mann warned. "The lesson is that a health threat in any part of the world can rapidly become a health threat to many or all."

Numerous other urgent global health challenges loom. In the 1980s and 1990s, more than 30 infectious diseases were identified in humans for the first time, including AIDS, Ebola, Hantavirus, and hepatitis C and E. In a case that aroused widespread concern in the U.S., health experts confirmed in October 1999, that at least five people in New York City and surrounding areas died from a new strain of the African West Nile virus, a rare mosquito-borne disease never before seen in the Western Hemisphere. They attribute the emergence of the disease to the steady rise in international trade and travel, concluding that it was transmitted either by an infected human who carried it into the country from abroad or via a smuggled exotic bird.

Environmental disruption is also a potent contributor to today's microbial migrations. According to WHO, "environmental changes have contributed in one way or another to the appearance of most if not all" of the newly emerging diseases. Changes in land use like deforestation or conversion of grasslands to agriculture that alter long-established equilibrium between microbes and their hosts are sometimes to blame. In other cases, changes in human behavior are the culprit, like careless disposal of food and beverage containers or car tires, which can create breeding sites for disease-carrying organisms such as mosquitoes. Movements of pathogens themselves or the organisms that carry them are sometimes the cause as well.

The Return of Cholera

An added problem is the reemergence of microbes thought to have been vanquished in some parts of the world. Cholera's reappearance in Latin America is a case in point. Until 1991, there had been no epidemic outbreaks of this deadly disease in this region for nearly a century. However, the disease erupted with a vengeance in Peru that year, ultimately infecting some 322,000 people and killing at least 2,900 of them. The outbreak was catastrophic for the country's economy, causing importers to ban Peruvian fish and fruit from their markets and tourists to avoid the country. All told, the economic costs to Peru's economy added up to $770,000,000—almost one-fifth of the country's normal annual export earnings.

The outbreak quickly spread beyond Peru, contaminating the water supply of every country on the continent except Paraguay and Uruguay before it gradually wound down two years later. Across the Americas, the disease infected more than 1,000,000 people and killed about 11,000 during the first half of the 1990s.

Scientists are trying to understand why cholera is reemerging with such force. A number of factors seem to be at work. One theory is that the cholera bacteria were discharged from the ballast water of ships arriving in Peruvian ports from South Asia. Poor sanitation undoubtedly played a major role, as cholera is often spread by contact with food or water that has been contaminated by human waste containing the bacteria. Another theory is that El Niño may have contributed to the outbreak by causing warmer ocean temperatures that encourage large blooms of plankton that can harbor the organism.

If El Niño was, in fact, a key piece of the puzzle, the cholera epidemic of the early 1990s was likely just a harbinger. Scientists project that climate change will lead to a surge in infectious ailments by increasing the range of disease-carrying organisms and inducing a growing number of extreme weather events such as floods and hurricanes, which tend to leave epidemics in their wake. "There are strong indications that a disturbing change in disease patterns has begun and that global warming is contributing to them," warns Paul Epstein, associate director of Harvard Medical School's Center for Health and the Global Environment. Already, dengue fever and malaria appear to be expanding their reach northward into cooler climates. Locally contracted cases of malaria have been reported in recent years in Florida, Georgia, Texas, Virginia, New York, New Jersey, Michigan, and Ontario, Canada. The record number of extreme weather events experienced in 1998 exacted a heavy toll on human health. Epstein reports that major flooding in East Africa led to large increases in the incidence of malaria, Rift Valley fever, and cholera; delayed monsoons in Southeast Asia contributed to wildfires that caused widespread respiratory ailments; and Central American nations slammed by Hurricane Mitch experienced an increase in cholera, dengue fever, and malaria.

Global Interdependence

With the global interdependence of human and ecological health creating frightening vulnerabilities, it is generating an imperative for countries to work together to confront shared perils. Faced with raging transcontinental epidemics of cholera and plague during the mid 19th century, European governments held 12 International Sanitary Conferences between 1851 and World War I which forged international health agreements covering issues such as quarantines, trade restrictions, and procedures for disease notification and inspection. In 1946, these and later efforts culminated in the creation of the World Health Organization, which has had a number of important successes, perhaps most notably the eradication of smallpox in 1977.

This system provides a firm foundation on which to build the new biological controls that are needed to protect people and ecosystems from the introduction of disruptive exotic diseases. Although economic globalization dominated headlines at the close of the 20th century, ecological integration may wind up posing even greater challenges for international cooperation in the decades ahead.

Tracking an Epidemic

BY JOSEPH B. MCCORMICK AND SUSAN FISHER-HOCH

The Centers for Disease Control and Prevention (CDC), headquartered in Atlanta, Georgia, is the chief government agency responsible for tracking and controlling epidemics and outbreaks (small epidemics) of infectious disease in the United States. Its Special Pathogens branch handles some of the most fearsome of these diseases. In 1996, when Joseph B. McCormick and his wife and fellow epidemiologist, Susan Fisher-Hoch wrote the memoir from which this excerpt was taken, McCormick was head of the CDC's Special Pathogens branch. The excerpt describes the first epidemic that McCormick investigated after joining the CDC; an outbreak of sore throats that he traced to contaminated potato salad at a Fourth of July picnic. He used the same basic epidemiological methods to track this homely cluster of illnesses that he and Fisher-Hoch would later apply in distant parts of the world as they followed the course of far deadlier ailments such as Ebola and Lassa fevers.

I arrived at the Centers for Disease Control and Prevention's (CDC) Atlanta, Georgia, headquarters in July 1973, just in time to begin the courses for incoming EIS (Epidemic Intelligence Service) officers. I would be replacing an outgoing officer named David Fraser, who was returning to the University of Pennsylvania to complete his fellowship in Infectious Diseases. I was assigned to the Special Pathogens Branch of the Division of Bacterial Diseases and was enrolled in the EIS course. That vital preparation is supposed to last a month, but, barely a week into the course, while I was attending a lecture, Roger Feldman, chief of Special Pathogens, walked in to seek me out. Now, Roger is a big man with a deep rumbling voice—a difficult guy to ignore. He located me, gave me a brisk tap on the shoulder, and said,

Joseph B. McCormick and Susan Fisher-Hoch, *Level 4: Virus Hunters of the CDC.* Atlanta, GA: Turner Publishing, 1996. Copyright © 1996 by Joseph B. McCormick. Reproduced by permission.

"I'm going to send you to Parker, Arizona, to an Indian reservation. There's a report that they have an epidemic of sore throats there. It could be streptococcal disease [caused by a common type of bacteria], but we're not sure."

"When do I leave?" I asked, trying to suppress my excitement at such an early opportunity to get into the field, even if the affliction was nothing more exotic than sore throats.

"You need to leave this afternoon," Roger said.

It was then nearly ten o'clock in the morning.

On-the-Job Training

Each year, one or two students would be pulled out of the EIS class to undertake an assignment because an emergency situation had arisen that demanded the presence of an investigator—any investigator—in the field immediately. Experience, if you didn't have it already, was something you acquired as you hit the ground running.

I was elated; couldn't believe my luck. My first epidemic sounded fantastic. An epidemic of sore throats—in the middle of summer! All I was told was that the victims had attended a Fourth of July picnic. At this stage of my professional preparation, I didn't even know that it is possible to get a sore throat from a food-borne infection.

I discovered that, in the enduring tradition of EIS, the first thing you have to do is become an instant expert. You have to get your hands on everything you can find on the subject and read it, for the most part en route to the site of the outbreak. Of course, you have to find real experts to brief you, too. However obscure a disease is, there is usually someone at CDC who knows about it. Mostly, though, you have to rely on yourself. You need to have an instinct for finding and absorbing information. Then you have to know how to use it sensibly. Although your immediate supervisor is someone who has done it before, and who knows most of the tricks, each epidemic is a little different, with its own twists and dilemmas, and it is up to you to solve them, but, more than that, to learn something new.

Tools of the Trade

Once you've gathered what you need to become an instant expert, your next step is to scramble around to collect the materials you'll need for the investigation: swabs, vials, syringes, sterilized packets of silicon gel for collecting cultures of strep, and so on. In the confusion, it's all you can do to remember to take a few pairs of clean socks and extra underwear along with you. On no account can you leave without an EPI 1 in your hand. This piece of paper constitutes your marching orders. Among other things, it confirms that the relevant state or local health agency has requested the assistance of CDC. As a federal agency, CDC must obtain the state's permission to initiate an investigation in its jurisdiction. The EPI 1 also specifies the individuals in the state health department you need to contact as soon as you get to where you're going. Once you reach your destination, you must first establish lines of communication with CDC in Atlanta, so that you'll have someone available twenty-four hours a day to answer questions and help you make decisions. The essence of the training is learning on the job, backed by extensive experienced support and supervision.

As a raw EIS officer, you're always wondering about whether you're adequately prepared. Questions constantly weigh upon your mind. Can I find the source of this disease? What can I do to stop this epidemic? Will I manage to get the correct data so I can completely define the problem and come up with the solution to it? Will I obtain cooperation from the state and local people I have to work with?

A Suspicious Picnic

A representative from the Arizona State Health Department was on hand to meet me in Phoenix. He told me that he'd be accompanying me to Parker, which was located about a hundred miles away, not far from the California border, and that he'd provide me with any assistance he could. Parker was a small town, but it was important because it served as a commercial hub for several nearby Indian reservations. The night of my arrival, I met with the physician who ran the small clinic on the reservation. He filled me in as much as he could. His story was straightforward: it began with a large Fourth of July picnic. Naturally, there was plenty of good food and beer. Then, a few days later, many of the picnickers—but not all—came down with severe streptococcal sore throats. The physician had seen many of the patients and had deduced that the one thing they had in common was that picnic. My job was to figure out why attending a picnic had put them at such risk, and then determine what I could do to stop any further cases from occurring. In theory, it sounded simple enough. But in practice?

I would soon find out.

In the articles I'd read on board the plane, I came across a report of an outbreak that had reminded me of this one. About a decade before, several people had developed sore throats after eating food contaminated with a certain strain of the streptococcus bacteria. This bacterium is the most common cause of sore throats. What made this particular infection serious, however, was that individuals, especially children, often go on to develop grave complications. Strep has been known to lead to rheumatic heart disease, kidney failure, severe skin conditions, and arthritis. Though these complications had rarely been reported in association with an epidemic, the possibility was worrying. I would have to move fast.

Bugs and People

An outbreak investigation is very much like the investigation of a crime. It consists of detective work, following hunches, and carefully collecting evidence. In epidemiology, however, the criminal is the bug. Find the bug. And then find how it got to its human hosts. The bug's motive? Making a lot more bugs, I guess.

But it's not just bugs that you're dealing with. You have to deal with people, especially the victims. It requires some effort to explain to them what you're doing, and then to convince them to cooperate. Fortunately, that wasn't a problem in Parker. Here, people were clearly concerned about the outbreak, and not the least concerned were those individuals who had been responsible for organizing the event. This was my first time on a Native American reservation, and it was turning into an important learning experience. To elicit information, I needed to work through a certain hierarchy of authority to insure that I didn't offend any of the leaders or elders. I was fortunate in having already learned the importance of this in African villages.

Asking Questions

I decided that this investigation needed to be done according to the book—what is called a case control study: This is a scientific method used by epidemiologists to discover the most important differences between those people who did become sick and those who did not. If you can determine these differences—particularly when it comes to food-borne outbreaks—you are usually close to pinpointing the cause or the route of infection. So I divided people who had been to the picnic into two groups: "cases" (people who had had sore throats) and "controls" (people who had not had sore throats).

Okay, now that I had my subjects, I had to figure out what to ask them. So I prepared a questionnaire. It had to be carefully worded, in order to elicit answers that were clearly in the category of yes or no. Basically, I was fishing for clues. Nonetheless, there was a certain logic to the questions. Some of them were obvious: Did you go to the picnic? Did you eat this dish, that dish, or the other dish? Did you drink this beverage or that one?

The investigator must be very careful in the way questions are phrased, so that they help people think clearly and insure accurate answers. It's easy to reach the wrong conclusions in investigations like the one I was conducting in Arizona. People tend to forget, or they may give a false answer in an effort to say what they believe is expected of them. There are certain things you tell the doctor, and other things you don't think he wants you to say. At the same time, I had to take specimens. This can only be done with the consent of the subjects, and it often required me to exercise all my powers of persuasion. In this particular outbreak, the obvious specimen was a throat swab. Once I was able to collect my swabs, I put them in special transport packets with silica gel in them. The gel would keep the bacterium alive until it reached the labs at CDC. There the specimens would be spread on special plates of agar jelly, which is rich with nutrients. If the strep was there, it would grow into round, grayish piles of organisms surrounded by transparent halos in the agar. Subsequent tests would tell us exactly what kind of strep we were dealing with.

Tracking Leftovers

I set about going from house to house, talking to people, marking my questionnaire, and sticking swabs down people's throats. I had no trouble confirming that the picnic had been the one common denominator. However, my case control study allowed me to pick up another crucial clue. All those who became sick had eaten one particular dish at the picnic: potato salad.

Now I had to find that potato salad—if there was any left.

My door-to-door inquiries turned up information that there were leftovers from the picnic. Next question: Who had them?

This required a survey—with surprisingly intimate questions. Then I had to ask permission to go rummaging in people's fridges and freezers. After locating samples of several of the picnic dishes in a freezer belonging to the community center at the reservation, I very carefully packed up this precious evidence and dispatched it back to CDC to see if the lab could culture the guilty streptococcus from it.

Sorting by Computer

After spending a week in Parker, I was ready to return to Atlanta for the second half of the investigation, which would continue in the lab. In the days before the personal computer, to obtain the statistical results of the questionnaire and other investigation inquiries, I had to enter all my data on punch cards. On the sixth floor of the CDC was an IBM machine known as a card sorter. It operated exclusively on a Yes/No answer system and sorted cards based on where holes had been punched in them. Although the machine was able to process each operation rather rapidly, it required a huge number of operations to arrive at an answer. Holes are punched in cards if the answer was yes, and left alone if the answer was no. The yes cards would then be separated into one pile, and the no cards in another. But if there are several levels to sort for, then the process of determining an answer grows progressively more difficult. If, for example, I wanted to find out whether all of the women who'd eaten potato salad had become ill compared to the men who had eaten it, I would have to sort the cards for all people who ate potato salad, then for all of the females and males. Then I would have to sort those cards for the females who ate potato salad and were ill. Cards would end up strewn all over the place. The whole business was very tedious. Nowadays, we put the information directly into a computer, enter a few instructions, and obtain the answers in a few seconds.

The Final Word

The lab had the final word: the potato salad harbored the culprit. Definitely strep. Apparently, after the potato salad was prepared, it had been left in large containers in the refrigerator, but because it took some time for the cold to penetrate the container, the center of the food remained warm for several hours—the perfect spot for bacteria contamination to live. It appeared that whoever had mixed the salad had been infected with strep. Because this person had not taken adequate food preparation precautions, the strep had got into the salad. The bacteria were just as happy about being in the warm center of the container, even in a refrigerator, as they would later be resting in the back of their host's throat.

So we prepared a report, an EPI II, to the health authorities in Parker, in which we described earlier recommendations to dispose of the frozen potato salad, and to be certain that individuals were appropriately treated with penicillin if suspected to harbor the organism in their throats. These measures were enough: the outbreak stopped, and no further cases occurred. I returned to my EIS course, but it was the Parker outbreak that provided me with the most practical foundation of my training in the scientific methods of epidemiology. It wouldn't be long before I would find myself searching for rats in Nigeria, surveying Sudanese villagers for incidences of Lassa [Fever], and asking patients about injections they'd received from general practitioners in Pakistan. No matter what situations I would face in the future, the basic methods at my disposal were those I learned tracking down suspect potato salad in a small southwestern town.

Disastrous Epidemics

The Plague of Athens

By Thucydides

The Greek historian Thucydides, who lived from about 460 to 400 B.C., is known for his objectivity and analysis of relationships between cause and effect in history. He began his career as a general in the city-state of Athens, but after being exiled for his loss of a key battle in the Peloponnesian War, fought between Athens and Sparta from 431 to 404 B.C., he turned to writing a history of the war. In Book II of this history he describes a mysterious epidemic that devastated Athens in 430 B.C., during the early years of the war, killing one-third of the city's people and all but destroying its fabled civilization. His account is perhaps the first to describe a major epidemic in detail. Historians still debate about what disease the "Plague of Athens" may have been; possibilities include measles, smallpox, or some type of infection that no longer exists.

I n the first days of summer [of 430 B.C.] the Lacæmonians and the allies, with two-thirds of their forces as before, invaded Attica [Greece], under the command of Archidamus, son of Zeuxidamus, king of Lacedæmon, and sat down and laid waste the country. Not many days after their arrival in Attica the plague first began to show itself among the Athenians. It was said that it had broken out in many places previously in the neighbourhood of Lemnos and elsewhere; but a pestilence of such extent and mortality was nowhere remembered. Neither were the physicians at first of any service, ignorant as they were of the proper way to treat it, but they died themselves the most thickly, as they visited the sick most often; nor did any human art succeed any better. Supplications in the temples, divinations, and so forth were found equally futile, till the overwhelming nature of the disaster at last put a stop to them altogether.

Thucydides, *History of the Peloponnesian War*, translated by Richard Crawley. New York: E.P. Dutton, 1910.

Start of the Plague

It first began, it is said, in the parts of Ethiopia [in East Africa]
above Egypt, and thence descended into Egypt and Libya and
into most of the king's country. Suddenly falling upon Athens, it
first attacked the population in Piræus [a nearby port city],—
which was the occasion of their saying that the Peloponnesians
had poisoned the reservoirs, there being as yet no wells there—
and afterwards appeared in the upper city, when the deaths became much more frequent. All speculation as to its origin and its
causes, if causes can be found adequate to produce so great a dis-
turbance, I leave to other writers, whether lay or professional; for
myself, I shall simply set down its nature, and explain the symptoms by which perhaps it may be recognised by the student, if it
should ever break out again. This I can the better do, as I had the
disease myself, and watched its operation in the case of others.

Course of the Disease

That year then is admitted to have been otherwise unprecedent-
edly free from sickness; and such few cases as occurred all deter-
mined in this. As a rule, however, there was no ostensible cause;
but people in good health were all of a sudden attacked by violent heats in the head, and redness and inflammation in the eyes,
the inward parts, such as the throat or tongue, becoming bloody
and emitting an unnatural and fetid breath. These symptoms were
followed by sneezing and hoarseness, after which the pain soon
reached the chest, and produced a hard cough. When it fixed in
the stomach, it upset it; and discharges of bile of every kind
named by physicians ensued, accompanied by very great distress.
In most cases also an ineffectual retching followed, producing violent spasms, which in some cases ceased soon after, in others
much later. Externally the body was not very hot to the touch,
nor pale in its appearance, but reddish, livid, and breaking out into
small pustules and ulcers. But internally it burned so that the patient could not bear to have on him clothing or linen even of the
very lightest description; or indeed to be otherwise than stark
naked. What they would have liked best would have been to
throw themselves into cold water; as indeed was done by some
of the neglected sick, who plunged into the rain-tanks in their
agonies of unquenchable thirst; though it made no difference
whether they drank little or much. Besides this, the miserable
feeling of not being able to rest or sleep never ceased to torment

them. The body meanwhile did not waste away so long as the distemper was at its height, but held out to a marvel against its ravages; so that when they succumbed, as in most cases, on the seventh or eighth day to the internal inflammation, they had still some strength in them. But if they passed this stage, and the disease descended further into the bowels, inducing a violent ulceration there accompanied by severe diarrhæa, this brought on a weakness which was generally fatal. For the disorder first settled in the head, ran its course from thence through the whole of the body, and even where it did not prove mortal, it still left its mark on the extremities; for it settled in the privy parts [genitals], the fingers and the toes, and many escaped with the loss of these, some too with that of their eyes. Others again were seized with an entire loss of memory on their first recovery, and did not know either themselves or their friends.

But while the nature of the distemper was such as to baffle all description, and its attacks almost too grievous for human nature to endure, it was still in the following circumstance that its difference from all ordinary disorders was most clearly shown. All the birds and beasts that prey upon human bodies, either abstained from touching them (though there were many lying unburied), or

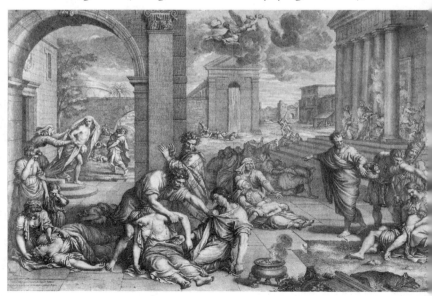

The Plague of Athens, depicted here, devastated the city of Athens in 430 B.C., killing one-third of its population.

died after tasting them. In proof of this, it was noticed that birds of this kind actually disappeared; they were not about the bodies, or indeed to be seen at all. But of course the effects which I have mentioned could best be studied in a domestic animal like the dog.

A Stricken Society

Such then, if we pass over the varieties of particular cases, which were many and peculiar, were the general features of the distemper. Meanwhile the town enjoyed an immunity from all the ordinary disorders; or if any case occurred, it ended in this. Some died in neglect, others in the midst of every attention. No remedy was found that could be used as a specific; for what did good in one case, did harm in another. Strong and weak constitutions proved equally incapable of resistance, all alike being swept away, although dieted with the utmost precaution. By far the most terrible feature in the malady was the dejection which ensued when any one felt himself sickening, for the despair into which they instantly fell took away their power of resistance, and left them a much easier prey to the disorder; besides which, there was the awful spectacle of men dying like sheep, through having caught the infection in nursing each other. This caused the greatest mortality. On the one hand, if they were afraid to visit each other, they perished from neglect; indeed many houses were emptied of their inmates for want of a nurse: on the other, if they ventured to do so, death was the consequence. This was especially the case with such as made any pretensions to goodness: honour made them unsparing of themselves in their attendance in their friends' houses, where even the members of the family were at last worn out by the moans of the dying, and succumbed to the force of the disaster. Yet it was with those who had recovered from the disease that the sick and the dying found most compassion. These knew what it was from experience, and had now no fear for themselves; for the same man was never attacked twice—never at least fatally. And such persons not only received the congratulations of others but themselves also, in the elation of the moment, half entertained the vain hope that they were for the future safe from any disease whatsoever.

Desperate Acts

An aggravation of the existing calamity was the influx from the country into the city, and this was especially felt by the new arrivals. As there were no houses to receive them, they had to be lodged at the hot season of the year in stifling cabins, where the mortality raged without restraint. The bodies of dying men lay one upon another, and half-dead creatures reeled about the streets and gathered round all the fountains in their longing for water. The sacred places also in which they had quartered themselves were full of corpses of persons that had died there, just as they were; for as the disaster passed all bounds, men, not knowing what was to become of them, became utterly careless of everything, whether sacred or profane. All the burial rites before in use were entirely upset, and they buried the bodies as best they could. Many from want of the proper appliances, through so many of their friends having died already had recourse to the most shameless sepultures: sometimes getting the start of those who had raised a pile [of wood on which a body was to be cremated] they threw their own dead body upon the stranger's pyre and ignited it; sometimes they tossed the corpse which they were carrying on the top of another that was burning and so went off.

Nor was this the only form of lawless extravagance which owed its origin to the plague. Men now coolly ventured on what they had formerly done in a corner, and not just as they pleased, seeing the rapid transitions produced by persons in prosperity suddenly dying and those who before had nothing succeeding to their property. So they resolved to spend quickly and enjoy themselves, regarding their lives and riches as alike things of a day. Perseverance in what men called honour was popular with none, it was so uncertain whether they would be spared to attain the object; but it was settled that present enjoyment, and all that contributed to it, was both honourable and useful. Fear of gods or law of man there was none to restrain them. As for the first, they judged it to be just the same whether they worshipped them or not, as they saw all alike perishing; and for the last, no one expected to live to be brought to trial for his offences, but each felt that a far severer sentence had been already passed upon them all and hung ever over their heads, and before this fell it was only reasonable to enjoy life a little.

Prophesies Remembered

Such was the nature of the calamity, and heavily did it weigh on the Athenians; death raging within the city and devastation without. Among other things which they remembered in their distress was, very naturally, the following verse which the old men said had long ago been uttered:

'A Dorian war shall come and with it death.'

So a dispute arose as to whether dearth [famine] and not death had not been the word in the verse; but at the present juncture, it was of course decided in favour of the latter; for the people made their recollection fit in with their sufferings. I fancy, however, that if another Dorian war should ever afterwards come upon us, and a dearth should happen to accompany it, the verse will probably be read accordingly. The oracle also which had been given to the Lacedæmonians was now remembered by those who knew of it. When the God was asked whether they should go to war, he answered that if they put their might into it, victory would be theirs, and that he would himself be with them. With this oracle events were supposed to tally. For the plague broke out so soon as the Peloponnesians invaded Attica, and never entering Peloponnese (not at least to an extent worth noticing), committed its worst ravages at Athens, and next to Athens, at the most populous of the other towns. Such was the history of the plague.

The Great Plague of London

By Thomas Vincent

Bubonic plague is most famous as the "Black Death" of medieval times, but epidemics of this disease swept through Europe and other parts of the world in many later eras as well. One of these epidemics, which struck Britain's capital in 1665, was known as the Great Plague of London. Perhaps the most detailed picture of this epidemic, excerpted here, was left by Thomas Vincent, a Puritan who saw the 1665 epidemic and the fire that brought a second wave of devastation to the city a year later as punishments from God. His account of these twin disasters, published in 1667, was called God's Terrible Voice in the City.

I t was in the year of our Lord 1665 that the plague began in our city of London, after we were warned by the great plague in Holland in the year 1664, and the beginning of it in some remote parts of our land in the same year, not to speak anything whether there was any signification and influence in the blazing star [probably a comet] not long before that appeared in the view of London, and struck some amazement upon the spirits of many. It was in the month of May that the plague was first taken notice of; our bill of mortality [list of deaths and their causes] did let us know but of three which died of the disease in the whole year before; but in the beginning of May the bill tells us of nine which fell by the plague—one in the heart of the city, the other eight in the suburbs. This was the first arrow of warning that was shot from heaven amongst us, and fear quickly begins to creep upon people's hearts; great thoughts and discourse there is in the town about the plague, and they cast in their minds whither they should go if the plague should increase. Yet when the next week's bill signifieth to them the decrease from nine to three their minds are

Thomas Vincent, *God's Terrible Voice in the City*. New York: E.P. Dutton, 1908.

something appeased, discourse of that subject cools, fears are hushed, and hopes take place that the black cloud did but threaten and give a few drops; but the wind would drive it away. But when in the next bill the number of the dead by the plague is mounted from three to fourteen, and in the next to seventeen, and in the next to forty-three, and the disease begins so much to increase and disperse, sinners begin to be startled.

Sudden Death

The plague is so deadly, it kills where it comes without mercy; it kills, I had almost said *certainly*; very few do escape, especially upon its first entrance and before its malignity be spent. Few are touched by it but they are killed by it, and it kills *suddenly*. As it gives no warning before it comes, suddenly the arrow is shot which woundeth unto the heart, so it gives little time for preparation before it brings to the grave. Under other diseases men may linger out many weeks and months, under some divers [numerous] years; but the plague usually killeth within, a few days, sometimes within a few hours after its first approach, though the body were never so strong and free from disease before.

Now [June] the citizens of London are put to a stop in the career of their trade [conduct of normal business]; they begin to fear whom they converse withal and deal withal, lest they should have come out of infected places. Now roses and other sweet flowers wither in the gardens, are disregarded in the markets, and people dare not offer them to their noses lest with their sweet savour that which is infectious should be attracted. Rue and wormwood [plants thought to have a protective effect] are taken into the hand, myrrh and zedoary into the mouth, and without some antidote few stir abroad in the morning. Now many houses are shut up where the plague comes and the inhabitants shut in, lest coming abroad they should spread the infection. It was very dismal to behold the red crosses, and read in great letters, "Lord, have mercy upon us," on the doors and, watchmen standing before them with halberts [weapons]; and such a solitude about those places, and people passing by them so gingerly and with such fearful looks, as if they had been lined with enemies in ambush that waited to destroy them.

The plague increaseth [July] and prevaileth exceedingly; the number of 470 which died in one week by the disease ariseth to 725 the next week, to 1089 the next, to 1843 the next, and to

2010 the next. Now the plague compasseth [surrounds] the walls of the city like a flood, and poureth in upon it. Now most parishes are infected, both without and within [the walls]; yea, there are not so many houses shut up by the plague as by the owners forsaking them for fear of it, and though the inhabitants be so exceedingly decreased by the departure of so many thousands, yet the number of dying persons doth increase fearfully. Now the countries

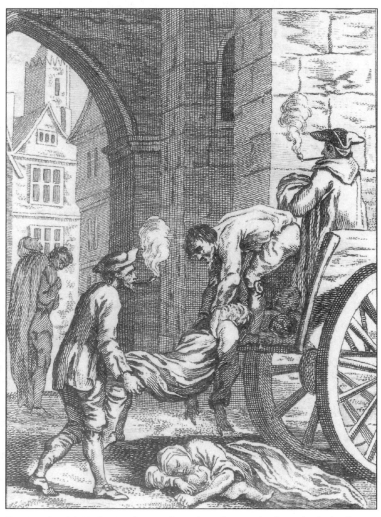

During the 1665 Great Plague of London, thousands of people died. The bodies of the dead were collected in carts and buried in huge pits.

keep guards lest infectious persons should from the city bring the disease unto them. Most of the rich are now gone, and the middle sort will not stay behind; but the poor are forced through poverty to stay and abide the storm. The very sinking fears they have had of the plague hath brought the plague and death upon many. Some by the sight of a coffin in the streets have fallen into a shivering, and immediately the disease has assaulted them; and Sergeant Death hath arrested them, and clapt to [shut] the doors of their houses upon them, from whence they have come forth no more till they have been brought to their graves.

It would be endless to speak of what we have seen and heard of some in their frenzy rising out of their beds and leaping about their rooms; others crying and roaring at their windows; some coming forth almost naked, and running into the streets. Strange things have others spoken and done when the disease was upon them; but it was very sad to hear of one who, being sick and alone, and, it is like [probable], frantic, burnt himself in his bed.

Silent Streets

In August how dreadful is the increase! Now the cloud is very black, and the storm comes down upon us very sharp. Now Death rides triumphantly on his pale horse through our streets, and breaks into every house almost where any inhabitants are to be found. Now people fall as thick as the leaves in autumn, when they are shaken by a mighty wind. Now there is a dismal solitude in London streets; every day looks with the face of a Sabbath-day [Sunday], observed with greater solemnity than it used to be in the city. Now shops are shut in, people rare and very few that walk about, insomuch that the grass begins to spring up in some places, and a deep silence almost in every place, especially within the walls; no prancing horses, no rattling coaches, no calling in customers, nor offering wares; no London cries sounding in the ears. If any voice be heard, it is the groans of dying persons, breathing forth their last, and the funeral knells of them that are ready to be carried to their graves. Now shutting up of visited houses (there being so many) is at an end, and most of the well are mingled among the sick, which otherwise would have got no help. Now in some places, where the people did generally stay, not one house in an hundred but what is infected; and in many houses half the family is swept away; in some the whole, from the eldest to the youngest: few escape but with the death of one or two. Never did so many husbands and wives die together; never did so many parents carry their children with them to the grave, and go together into the same house under earth, who had lived together in the same house upon it. Now the nights are too short to bury the dead: the whole day, though at so great a length, is hardly sufficient to light the dead that fall thereon into their graves. We could hardly go forth but we should meet many coffins, and see many with sores and limping in the streets.

Now [September] the grave doth open its mouth without measure. Multitudes! multitudes in the valley of the shadow of death, thronging daily into eternity. The churchyards now are stuffed so full with dead corpses that they are in many places swelled two or three feet higher than they were before, and new ground is broken up to bury the dead.

The "Spanish Flu" Epidemic of 1918

By Lynette Iezzoni

People think of the flu as more a nuisance than a disaster, but some strains of the influenza virus can be deadly. As documentary filmmaker Lynette Iezzoni explains, one strain produced the worst epidemic in U.S. history (it also affected many other countries). The epidemic, which began at a military barracks in Fort Riley, Kansas, in spring 1918, just as World War I was ending, sickened some 25 million Americans and killed 675,000 of them within just a few months. Less than a year after its beginning, it stopped as mysteriously as it had started. In this excerpt from her book Influenza 1918, *Iezzoni weaves together survivors' recollections to describe the breakdown of daily social life that the epidemic produced in American towns and cities.*

In Denver, Colorado, Katherine Anne Porter's flu led to delirium. Her fever became so high her hair turned white and fell out. Her lieutenant [fiancé] nursed her patiently, despite the shrill objections of her landlady. From [Porter's novella] "Pale Horse, Pale Rider":

> Miss Hobbe with her face all out of shape with terror was crying shrilly, "I tell you they must come for her now, or I'll put her on the sidewalk . . . I tell you, this is a plague, a plague, my God!"

> I lay back on the pillow and thought, I must give up, I can't hold out any longer. There was only that pain, only that room. There was only this one moment and it was a dream of time . . . "I'm not unconscious," I explained, "I know what I want to say." Then to my horror I heard myself babbling nonsense . . .

A terrible compelling pain ran through her veins like heavy fire. The stench of corruption filled her nostrils, the sweetish sickening smell of rotting flesh and pus. The smell of death was in her own body.

A Climate of Fear

All across the nation, men, women, and children were sick. For millions of Americans, life had become a painful, nightmarish ordeal. For the robust, those who remained standing, life had become nearly as surreal. All health seemed vanished from the world. The plague was everywhere. No city, no home, no family, no person was safe. Like the medieval Black Death, Spanish influenza was as implacable and ephemeral as fog, an oppressive, ghostly presence. According to schoolgirl Georgina Cragg, "the fear was so thick even a child could feel it." The rituals of community life—gossip over the pushcart, conversation by the fencepost, the games of children and the commerce of churches—all the discrete moments which, woven together, created the rich fabric of American life—were failing to occur. Even an act as simple and natural as shaking hands could invite the angel of death. People were afraid of each other. Neighbors vanished inside their homes. Life had been utterly disrupted.

In the Sardo's funeral home in Washington, D.C., the fear was palpable. Bill Sardo remembers:

> From the moment I got up in the morning to when I went to bed at night, I felt a constant sense of fear. We wore gauze masks. We were afraid to kiss each other, to eat with each other, to have contact of any kind. We had no family life, no school life, no church life, no community life. Fear tore people apart.

In Philadelphia, Susanna Turner's neighborhood had turned into a bleak, unwelcoming place.

> Neighbors weren't helping neighbors. No one was taking any chances. People became selfish. We lost our spirit of charity. Fear just withered the hearts of people.

Dan Tonkel of Goldsboro, North Carolina recalls:

> I felt like I was walking on eggshells. I was afraid to go out, to play with my playmates, my classmates, my

neighbors. I was almost afraid to breathe. I remember I
was actually afraid to breathe. People were afraid to talk
to each other. It was like—don't breathe in my face,
don't even look at me, because you might give me
germs that will kill me.

Life Comes to a Halt

The peaceful rhythms of small town life had been shattered.
Goldsboro's streets were deserted.

> Farmers stopped farming, merchants stopped selling.
> The county more or less just shut down. Everyone was
> holding their breath, waiting for something to happen.
> So many people were dying, we could hardly count
> them. We never knew from one day to another who
> was going to be next on the death list.

All across America, community life was grinding to a halt.
Schools and factories closed. Churches, libraries, and private clubs
locked their doors. Courts recessed. Newspapers folded or simply stopped printing ("Don't expect the next *Courier* until you
see it," one wrote). Government services failed. Policemen were
sick, as were firemen, trash collectors, and trolley drivers. Garbage
remained dumped on city streets. No [telephone] "Operator" answered to place a call. Essentials, like food and coal, became
scarce: merchants were sick or fearful. Steel and coal production
faltered, as did the machinery and business of war. Riveting guns
fell silent in naval shipyards. Production lines halted in munitions
factories. Army camps were paralyzed. Army Chief of Staff Pay-
ton March cabled General Pershing in France, "Influenza not
only stopped all draft calls in October, but practically all training."
The business of war and the commerce of daily life in America were both falling victim to the plague. Captain George T.
Palmer of the Army Sanitary Corps advised, "Abandon the uni-
versal practice of shaking hands. Substitute some other less intimate method of salutation." Americans were cautioned against
leaving home, against riding trolleys, against checking a book out
from the library, against "slacking" with their masks. The magazine *Science* reported 119 daily opportunities for infection, from
turning a doorknob to paying a grocery bill. Official and unof-
ficial advice poured forth, intensifying the dread and panic, feed-
ing a mad rumor-mill of weird, improbable cures and contradic-

tory advice. Castor oil was advisable. Castor oil was not advisable. Fresh air and exercise were the ticket; it was better to stay home and rest. No one knew what to do.

Poisonous Rumors

Widespread rumors of a German plot intensified. Some claimed Bayer aspirin (whose original patent had been German) was filled with poisoned germs. The Public Health Service was compelled to investigate the claims, claims which were disproved. Had German spies infiltrated the Army Medical Corps and spread Spanish influenza through hypodermic shots? Had the spies been discovered and executed by firing squad? Rumors persisted, despite strenuous denials by the Surgeon General of the Army, Brigadier General Charles Richard: "There have been no medical officers or nurses or anyone else executed at camps in the United States." Nevertheless, many Americans continued to blame the Germans for Spanish influenza. One patriot declared,

> Let the curse be called the German plague. Let every child learn to associate what is accursed with the word German not in the spirit of hate but in the spirit of contempt born of the hateful truth which Germany has proved herself to be.

The moral fabric of America was unraveling, bit by bit. The foundations of American society—education, law, religion—all seemed in jeopardy. Even the institution of family was shaken. Influenza was the invisible enemy. The visible enemy, the clear and obvious source of danger, was one's fellow man—especially the members of one's family. Many families, out of necessity, lack of options, love, compassion, or feelings of dutiful responsibility, persisted in what was, at the time, a familiar exercise: to nurse one's own. Because of the breadth of the catastrophe, women, society's traditional "ministering angels," were joined in great numbers by men like Katherine Anne Porter's gentle lieutenant. . . . For other families, however, the silent, savage intruder which had invaded their home, their dinner table, and their beds exposed or aggravated existing tensions. Often, answering a call reporting the terminally ill, health authorities would arrive at the scene and find no one home but the dying—the families had deserted them. In Minneapolis, a hundred homeless children, some sick, some not, were found hiding out on the streets, their parents vanished.

Stealing Coffins

In West Philadelphia, every hour brought another knock on the door of the Donohues' funeral home from people bearing their dead. Increasingly, the grim pandemonium contained a bizarre irony. Desperate to provide dignity for their deceased relatives, people were stealing caskets. The Donohues were forced to hire men to guard their small stash of coffins. Michael Donohue explains:

> Normally, stealing a casket would be inconceivable. It would be equated with grave robbing. But in October 1918, the influenza epidemic changed people's minds about what they would do, how they would act. People were desperate. They felt they had no alternative, there was no place for them to turn. These were nice people, people who wouldn't have done this otherwise. These were our neighbors, our friends, and for some of them, stealing a casket was the only way they could see to provide for their loved one.

Season of Death

Autumn had truly become the season of death.

The numbers were staggering. In the state of New York, 500,000 people were sick with influenza and related pneumonia. In Pennsylvania, 350,000 were sick; in New Jersey, 100,000; Connecticut, 110,000; Virginia, 220,000; Ohio, 150,000; Nebraska, 40,000; Minnesota, 35,000; and California, 40,000. In Venice, California, the Al. G. Barnes Circus underwent a mandatory "fumigation." Lions, elephants, and ponies, as well as trapeze artists, contortionists, and the "Albino Girl," were sprayed with a foul mixture of coal tar and formaldehyde. In Chicago, October 17 became known as "Black Thursday": 381 people died and 1,200 fell sick. The city ran out of hearses. Passenger trolleys were draped in black and used to collect bodies. Signs were posted:

> There shall be no public funerals held in Chicago over any body dead from any disease or cause whatsoever. No wakes or public gatherings of any kind shall be held in connection with these bodies. No one except adult relatives and friends not to exceed ten persons in addition to the undertaker, undertaker's assistants, minister, and

necessary drivers shall be permitted to attend any funeral. No dead body shall be taken into any church or chapel for funeral services in connection with such body.

Brutal Laws

Laws veered towards the brutal. Chicago's Health Commissioner, Dr. John Dill Robertson, turned his considerable wrath against spitters and "openfaced sneezers." He ordered the police, "Arrest thousands, if necessary, to stop sneezing in public!" Only Reverend J.P. Brushingham of Chicago's Morals Commission noted a silver lining in the plague's dark cloud. In the month of October, Chicago's crime rate dropped by 43 percent.

Even New York's nervy, indomitable Royal Copeland was growing tense. Each day, 5,500 New Yorkers fell sick with influenza. On October 23, 851 people died: mortality figures which surpassed even those of Philadelphia. The Empire City and the Empire State had become the deadliest place in the nation. Health Commissioner Copeland, whose rambling and verbose Congressional oratories later earned him the nickname "General Exodus," lashed out at his fellow physicians. Sloppy morbidity and mortality reports were skewing the daily totals. Late or messy reports would be slapped with a five hundred dollar fine. State Commissioner of Health, Herman Biggs, joined in with a fine of his own: any person who coughed or sneezed in the state of New York without a handkerchief would pay five hundred dollars or spend a year in jail. Huge signs appeared on New York streets: "It is Unlawful to Cough and Sneeze." Five hundred "snifflers" were dragged into court. Spitters suffered a similar fate.

Orphaned Children

In Brooklyn, New York, six-year-old Michael Wind stood among his brothers and sisters.

> When my mother died of Spanish influenza, we were all gathered in one room, all six of us, from age two to age twelve. My father was sitting beside my mother's bed, head in his hands, sobbing bitterly. All my mother's friends were there, with tears of shock in their eyes. They were shouting at my father, asking why he hadn't called them, hadn't told them she was sick. She had been fine yesterday. How could this have happened?

The next morning, his father took Michael and his two younger brothers to the subway. He bought each child a Hershey bar. Michael Wind: "I knew then that something was wrong. My father couldn't afford such treats. Sure enough, we were on our way to an orphanage." Michael and his brothers were placed in the Brooklyn Hebrew Orphan Asylum. The Asylum was filled with six hundred boys and girls, most orphaned by the flu.

Bloody Death: Ebola Fever

BY NANCY GIBBS

Ebola fever, a virus-caused illness found (so far) chiefly in central Africa, has caused fewer than a thousand known deaths, but this article by Nancy Gibbs shows why it is one of the most dramatic of recently discovered, "emerging" epidemic diseases. Gibbs, a senior editor at Time *magazine, describes vividly how Ebola, one of a group of illnesses called hemorrhagic fevers because of the extensive internal bleeding they cause, makes "organs . . . melt" and "red-black sludge wiggle out of [a patient's] eyes." She recounts how health care workers from the World Health Organization, the U.S. Centers for Disease Control and Prevention, and other groups joined local people in responding to a deadly outbreak of Ebola centering on the city of Kikwit, in Zaire (now Democratic Republic of Congo), in April and May 1995.*

In the darkened doorway of an abandoned building, the medical team finds an empty coffin, waiting like carrion. One by one, neighbors explain, the family that lived there died. First the daughter, 18, went to the Kikwit 2 maternity hospital [in Zaire] in late March [1995] for a caesarean section. When she got home her incision began to bleed. Then her organs began to melt. The red–black sludge wiggled out of her eyes, her nose, her mouth. Soon her parents got sick. Her father, some villagers believe, died of horror: he told his wife that if she died, he would die too on the next Friday. And he did, followed by another daughter, then two sons, and a nurse who had helped tend them.

Two houses away, a new widow sits and watches the visitors making their way through town. Her husband, she quietly admits, also helped take care of the sick family. Then he died. She buried his body, but the mattress where he lay sick is still in the house. Dr. David Heymann of the World Health Organization [WHO] listens to her story, and his heart sinks. He knows as much about the lethal Ebola virus as anyone alive; he was part of the team that investigated the first recorded outbreak, also in Zaire, in 1976. Now he is leading the international brigade that has come to the city of Kikwit to battle the new emergency. "The virus is still loose, and it's spreading," he says. "If the mattress is warm and damp, and people go in and sleep on it, we're going to be in trouble." The villagers are terrified, and resigned. "It's useless for us to do anything," says a neighbor, Mbangu Fioti. "What can we do against this disease?"

For a while [in mid-May 1995] . . . it looked as though the outbreak might soon be brought under control. The plague police—medical teams dispatched by WHO in Geneva, the Centers for Disease Control and Prevention (CDC) in Atlanta and other public health groups—had set up an effective isolation ward at the main hospital in Kikwit, where the first case had been identified. Belgium's Doctors Without Borders (Medecins Sans Frontieres, or MSF) rushed in loads of gloves, gowns, masks and other essential equipment to restore hygiene to filthy clinics. But when the strike forces, aided by local medical students, fanned out through the countryside around Kikwit, trying to follow the path of the fever, it became clear that the danger was far from past.

The teams' job was to figure out who might have been infected already and to warn people at risk. At first doctors thought the victims could all be traced back to a 36-year-old lab technician named Kimfumu, who died at Kikwit's main hospital [in April 1995]. . . . But once they discovered the case of the woman infected even earlier at the Kikwit 2 maternity hospital, they realized the crisis was worse than they had imagined. "It's a huge epidemic," Heyman says of the previously unrecorded cases, "and it's got nothing to do with the main hospital." By [about May 22] . . . WHO doctors had counted 97 Ebola deaths, and the toll seemed certain to rise much higher. The only good news was that the disease had not yet spread—as far as anyone could tell—to the 4 million people of Kinshasa [the capital of Zaire], 250 miles to the west.

When the doctors descended on Kikwit 2, the only hint of hygiene was a torn garbage bag on the rusting operating table that clearly had not been changed for months. There were no lights, no running water; health workers collected rainwater from a cistern or went down to the river with buckets. Conditions were perfect for breeding a plague.

And there is more bad news. Since Kimfumu perished . . . no one has dared enter the thatched-roof hut where he lived. Mute children and frightened neighbors stare at the stick fence and whisper, as medical students arrive to search for the dead man's family and friends. Where is the cure, a man named Mola asks. A student explains that there is no cure; the only hope is prevention, staying away from the sick, not touching the body. Mola frowns. "I don't know what to say," he says. His father has just died from the virus. "I am the one who helped him. I have already touched the body. And now you tell me I must avoid contact?"

Mola confirms a grim fact about how the disease has spread. Though the Ebola virus is not easily transmitted—it is passed by contact with blood and body fluids—Zairian custom requires that preparation of a body for burial must include the handling of various organs. Health officials had hoped only family members were involved in the burial; from Mola and others they learn that friends help as well, which means even more people are in peril than the doctors had realized. "We are telling people of the enormous risks involved in doing this, and offering a safe and respectful form of burial with the aid of the Red Cross," says WHO spokesman Thomson Prentice. When the family insists on a traditional burial, he adds, "we are trying to tell families how to do so at the lowest possible risk. But it's really a tough fight."

As dedicated as the relief effort has been, Heyman realizes that it is not enough. He consults with local officials and orders that the teams of students tracking down possible victims be doubled. He wants bicycles, so the teams can travel more quickly, and more gowns, more rubber gloves, more masks to help protect families of the sick and workers in local clinics. He continually quizzes the students, to make sure they are asking the right questions and searching for the right clues.

He knows how hard their job is; their own friends and families are shunning them. "Even the taxis will not take us," says a pretty third-year student named Isabelle Lumbwe, 23. "Our friends say we should be quarantined." But the students are undaunted. "This is going to be our work," she says. "What kind of soldier are you if you flee the battle?"

The problem, the medical teams realize, is that since all the early cases were centered in hospitals, people are afraid to go to them. Officials try to spread the word that the main hospital, at least, is cleaner now, with better staff, supplies and hygiene. But whether out of fear or custom, the sick prefer to go home to die. Relief workers are finding eight, nine people living under the same roof with a potential Ebola patient. So teams of local workers fan out through the towns with bullhorns, describing symptoms, advising people of the risks and preparing pamphlets with pictures—designed for those who can't read—about how to care for the sick without catching the virus. The personnel are quickly engulfed by huge crowds of people desperate for information and reassurance.

Meanwhile, at the main hospital, a group of low, tin-roofed buildings painted sky blue in the center of town, Dr. Pierre Rollin, chief of the CDC's pathogenesis [disease origin] section, has restored some semblance of order since patients and workers fled the catastrophe. "When we arrived," he says, "it was very bad. People were vomiting; there was diarrhea and blood all over the floors and walls. The dead were lying among the living." Relatives who came to care for their loved ones walked in and out of isolation without protection.

Fully suited up in gowns, goggles and masks, Rollin's team went from bed to bed, picking up bodies off the floors. Workers then washed down the walls and floors and took the corpses to the morgue. The isolation ward was wrapped in a 6-ft. swath of gray plastic; at the entrance was a basin of disinfectant, so people would not carry the virus out on the soles of their shoes. A Belgian Jesuit missionary conducted last rites at a distance.

The staff now tries to teach caution: relatives are given masks and gowns and told to wash their hands before taking the gloves off. Only one family member is allowed to visit. "If I had a choice, I would prohibit it," admits Rollin, "but that's not possible here." The hospital has no kitchen, so the families provide the patients' meals. The staff is careful not to scare people off. "You can't hold patients against their will," says Heyman. "If we were to use force, then patients would be even less likely to come."

The situation is more desperate at the local clinics outside the city. Dr. Bele Okwo, an American-trained epidemiologist, is in charge of surveillance in the outlying villages. It is here that Zaire's poverty takes its most obvious toll. "We are so poor, we cannot take the necessary precautions," he says. "To maintain hygiene, you need funds, and we don't have them." Even WHO had no money in its budget for a quick-response team. When Heymann was summoned to Zaire, he begged the local pharmacies in Geneva for every gown and glove he could get his hands on.

For all the hard work of the Zairian doctors and students and the expertise offered by the international aid workers, the hardest job of all falls to the 26 local Red Cross workers. They drive through the villages in a bright orange Renault truck, picking up bodies and wrapping them in plastic as infected blood oozes everywhere. Unless the family dares claim a body, it is driven out of town to a mass grave. Until MSF arrived with protective gear, the Red Cross worked with bare hands; already three victims have died of the virus, and one more fell ill. . . . The gravediggers are pariahs. When they walk down the street, the children scatter. Their families have left them. Each day, in fact, frightened residents are abandoning anyone who gets sick, even from common illnesses. Parents are shunning their children. One day . . . a sickly looking young man sat in the middle of a soccer field, rocking back and forth. No one dared come near him.

AIDS in Zambia

BY JAN GOODWIN

*In this article, award-winning journalist and human rights activist Jan
Goodwin portrays the social devastation that the AIDS pandemic has
brought to the country of Zambia, in southern Africa, where one in every
four people is infected with the virus that causes the disease. Whole families have been wiped out, Goodwin says, and orphaned children roam the
streets or struggle to act as parents for younger siblings. Victims' sufferings
are made worse by the need to hide their illness in order to avoid ostracism from other members of the community. At the end of the article,
Goodwin offers hope by describing steps that some Zambians are taking
to control the epidemic. Goodwin edits the "On the Issues" column in*
Harper's Bazaar *and has also written several books, including* Price of
Honor, *which examines how Islamic extremism affects the lives of Mus-
lim women.*

The crowds outside the city mortuary start forming shortly
after daybreak. It's Sunday morning, a time in Lusaka,
Zambia, once devoted to observing the Sabbath, not
burying the dead.

As the sun rises, a line of traffic builds up, mostly pickups and
small trucks bringing mourners, pickaxes, and shovels. There's
sharp competition for gravediggers; the main cemeteries are full,
and even the new ones are running out of space. Shipping containers, used as makeshift coffin and wreath stores, clog the side-
walks. In this impoverished southern African country with a 60
percent unemployment rate, the only boom industry is death. But
a growing number of families, who've buried too many relatives,
can no longer afford shop-bought coffins and must construct
their own. One anguished father, too poor even to rent a vehicle
for a few hours, arrives on foot carrying a handcrafted pine box
for a child.

DON'T PANIC, GOD IS WITH YOU reads a sign above

one coffin store. Outside, a church choir sings a hymn: "Dance for the Lord, the world is at an end."

A Parade of Funerals

To Zambians, it may very well feel like the end of the world. In 2001, the country is 17 years into an HIV/AIDS pandemic. One in four of the 9.5 million population is infected, according to experts in Zambia, and in some areas it's risen to one in three. Teachers, doctors, nurses, and civil servants are dying as fast as replacements can be found. Banks now train two people for every job in the hope that one will survive. The largest medical institute in the country, Lusaka's University Teaching Hospital, has only 600 nurses—little more than a third of what it once had—yet its patient intake has never been higher.

Thirty-year-old Namukolo Phiri is burying her husband, Emmanuel. Thin and suffering from a raging fever, Phiri is herself already ill with AIDS symptoms, and she is six months pregnant with her fourth child. "Emmanuel had a very bad headache, then he died," she says, weeping and shivering on the cemetery ground as she watches family members dig her husband's grave. "He became sick and died just like his parents and my sister and brother." Her grief is made all the worse by fear of what will happen to her children.

As many as 1.5 million children in Zambia have lost one or both parents to AIDS—the highest rate, as a proportion of population, in the world, according to the United Nations. Talk to any Zambian, from government officials to the poorest villagers, and you learn they are raising the children of relatives who have died.

The problem is all the greater because Zambians are reluctant to accept that HIV is the cause of all the dying. The stigma of AIDS is so enormous here, survivors prefer to say that family members died from tuberculosis (TB) or meningitis, common AIDS-related conditions. Phiri believes that her sister and brother, as well as her parents-in-law, died of TB. Physicians encourage euphemism by falsifying death certificates, because they know that honesty means the surviving spouse and children may be shunned, even turned out of their homes. Often, the truth is withheld from AIDS patients themselves. HIV testing in Zambia is infrequent, and when it is done, medical personnel often don't inform patients they are positive because they claim it will distress them too much.

Pastor Simon Chileshe, who is presiding over Emmanuel's funeral service, is a little more direct: "If you plant ground nuts, you will harvest ground nuts, not oranges," he thunders. "This means we should not go about with other people's spouses. If we do, it will lead us to big problems like you see here."

Overburdened Adults, Orphaned Children

It is true that male promiscuity—long accepted, even expected, in Zambian culture—is a major contributing factor to the high HIV/AIDS rate. A study has shown that men who have extramarital sex partners and are therefore apt to contract sexually transmitted diseases (STDs) including HIV, are more likely to abuse their wives. The threat of physical violence and the fear of abandonment, economically and physically, make it hard for women to negotiate the use of condoms, discuss fidelity, or leave relationships.

Phiri's eyes fill with tears again. "My husband repented his ways when we joined the Pentecostal Church," she says. "But he repented too late."

Women are likewise often powerless to avoid infecting their own children. Even a baby who manages to avoid contracting HIV in utero or during delivery has about a one in three chance of getting the virus from breast-feeding. Yet women continue to nurse, because formula is expensive, and any mother who feeds her child infant formula is assumed to be HIV positive and risks ostracism. Anti-AIDS drugs such as AZT [azidothymidine] or nevirapine, which can lower the risk of mother-to-child transmission by as much as 50 percent, are rarely available. And if they are, they only pose a further dilemma for the mother: The drug may let my baby live, but what happens to my child when I die of AIDS?

Obviously, HIV has caused an array of overlapping and intractable problems in Zambia—and much of the rest of Africa. But one look at the situation is all it takes to see that women, because of their central yet still largely vulnerable position in society, have come to bear the greatest share of the AIDS burden. . . .

A Government in Denial

Because denial holds such sway over the culture, Zambia has little in the way of a national HIV/AIDS education program. In Uganda, by contrast, the government has conducted a massive campaign bluntly explaining how to prevent the disease, and during the 1990s, infection rates dropped to 8 percent from a high of 18 percent. "Uganda has a model program for the world," says Sandra Thurman, former director of the U.S. White House Office of National AIDS Policy. Zambia's government, on the other hand, passive to the point of inertia, would appear to be a model of how not to handle the crisis. Life expectancy has dropped from 56 years to 37 in recent years, and observers believe it could reach as low as 30 by 2010.

Yet when a Dutch journalist presented photographs documenting the Zambian predicament at the international AIDS conference in Durban, South Africa, in 2000, the Zambian government's response was embarrassed outrage that they were publicized. That this is a crisis officials would prefer not be exposed appeared to be confirmed when *Bazaar*'s writer and photographer were arrested and held while reporting this story, although ultimately they were not charged. Similarly, government officials failed to keep appointments with *Bazaar* to discuss HIV/AIDS. Perhaps they realized there was little they could talk about. Zambia's National AIDS Council, which was finally created in the spring of 2000, was still not functioning six months later. The one staff member and two clerks in the office seemed not to know where to begin, no one knew what the budget was, and the only thing on the agenda was an apparently never-ending debate as to who the council members should be.

When the son of former president Kenneth Kuanda died of AIDS, the reaction in government circles was: "How could the family admit it?"

A Teenage "Mother"

For 19-year-old Rachel Musonda, who lives in the Copperbelt mining region in the north of the country, the time from 1997 to 2000 has been a nightmare, as first her father, then her mother, and then her three older siblings died of AIDS. With each new casualty, Musonda, who was forced to drop out of high school to nurse her parents and who has no skills or financial means, has been left with more children to raise. At 15, she had no choice but to become mother and father to her six younger siblings, then aged from 13 down to one year. With the subsequent deaths of her two older sisters and brother, and their spouses, she had to take on three more children, bringing the total to nine, because there was nowhere else for them to go.

Musonda, with her slight frame and shy smile, looks younger than 19, though the shadows under her large eyes and the constant plucking at the hem of her skirt as she talks attest to the stress she is under. She is particularly concerned about Diana, her sister Vivian's child, who was only eight months old when her mother died and may well be infected with HIV. Now five, Diana is still not strong. But even if she were tested for HIV, there are no drug therapies available to treat her.

Anti-AIDS medications cost $10,000 to $15,000 a year, more than the vast majority of Africans earn in a lifetime. "AIDS drugs are a nonstarter for this country," confirms Peter McDermott, former UNICEF [United Nations International Children's Emergency Fund, now United Nations Children's Fund] representative to Zambia. The government is obliged by International Monetary Fund guidelines to spend more on international-debt servicing than it does on education and health combined. Consequently, the country's budget for health care is a pitiful $6 to $8 per person per year, and that sum includes the cost of hospitals and treating other rampant health problems such as malaria.

The U.S. offered a $1 billion loan in 2000 to the worst-hit sub-Saharan African nations, including Zambia, to buy AIDS drugs from American companies, but many governments turned it down because they could not afford to increase their annual debt-servicing commitments. And even the discounted price of $2000 a year per patient is still a fantastical sum for Zambians, representing as it does an average of nearly seven years' income for the 40 percent who are fortunate enough to be employed.

Further complicating the issue, anti-AIDS medications can cause serious side effects, including bone-marrow suppression [resulting in loss of blood cells], which requires strict monitoring. And because diarrhea and vomiting are a common problem for patients on AIDS protocols, medications must be taken on a strictly observed schedule around meals. In Zambia, the reality is that many people can eat only when food is available. And that is increasingly becoming only once every several days.

No Money, No Food

When we meet, Musonda and the children she cares for have not eaten for two days. "The younger ones are not as big as they should be because they don't get enough food," she says. Stunted growth is common in Zambia, where more than 50 percent of children are chronically malnourished. When it achieved independence from Britain in 1964, this country was the third-richest in Africa, but today, after nearly three decades of Marxism and mismanagement, it is one of the poorest. Critics of President Frederick Chiluba, a former trade unionist, charge that he spends more time worrying about the war in neighboring Congo than he does fighting the one that HIV/AIDS is waging on his own country.

Musonda's family eats only when she can sell a few flour-and-water drop-scones (a sort of small pancake), and she can make these only if there is money to purchase the flour. Few of her fellow neighbors in Chimwemwe Compound (a Copperbelt shantytown) can afford the luxury of buying her scones. Musonda sells them for a pittance, and she is lucky to make a few cents a day, which in Zambia doesn't stretch to buy both the next bag of flour and enough nshima (maize meal, a Zambian staple similar to porridge) to feed a family of 10.

When she does have flour, Musonda rises at dawn to make the scones over a wood fire in the hardscrabble yard. She tries to ignore her own hunger pangs as she cooks, and gives the burned fragments to the younger children. "They fight over the little pieces, watching me like baby birds waiting to be fed," she says. She looks off into the distance as she reminisces: "I try not to remember the dishes my mother used to make, like her chicken." The 10 of them haven't eaten meat of any kind since her parents died. Even if she had the money, she wouldn't buy it, she says. "For the price of a chicken, which lasts only one meal, I can buy nshima, and maybe a few vegetables, for a whole week."

She worries all the time about food, clothes, the children's health. "Now, when I need my parents for advice, they're not here," she says. "I get so tired trying to do everything alone." Despite her exhaustion, and the lack of running water, the two-room home is spotless. The fence of rusting auto-body parts was erected by her father, who repaired cars for a living. In the yard, a dilapidated automobile sits where its tires have rotted into the ground. "My brother John wanted to repair it and earn a living as a driver," says Musonda, "but he died before he could start."

Inside, on the scrubbed table, the only decorative touches are two table mats embroidered by her sister Vivian shortly before her death. A closet in one corner contains a stack of shining metal plates and cooking pots, which along with four rickety chairs constitute the Musonda family's wealth today. Ten kids share four blankets. The other family blankets have been used as makeshift burial shrouds, and Musonda, who intended to be an elementary-school teacher until her education came to an abrupt halt, is unable to purchase replacements. There are no longer any beds. The four younger children sleep on a slab of discarded industrial foam rubber, the other six on the bare floor. In the winter, when temperatures sink to 40 [degrees] F. and wind whistles through the broken windows, and during the rainy season, the children huddle at night to consolidate body warmth. The clothes her charges wear are either too small or threadbare from too much laundering. Shoes are a thing of the past.

Still, what hurts Musonda the most, and makes her tear up, is facing Sundays, when the family used to attend the Seventh-Day Adventist Church together. "People here always dress in their best to go to church," she says. "But the kids are now so ragged, they are too ashamed to go." . . .

Street Kids

Another growing factor in the spread of AIDS is the legion of street kids, often AIDS orphans, many of whom must turn to prostitution to survive, as the country has only a handful of orphanages. About 750,000 children, some as young as four, have already been forced onto the streets.

A visit to one of the few shelters for street kids in Lusaka, the Fountain of Hope drop-in center, reveals that the city is already full of child victims of the AIDS pandemic. The youngest children at the center were Betty Kabemba, four, and her six-year-old sister, Ruth, who survived on the streets for five months by begging before they were spotted by an outreach worker. The girls said their father left for South Africa in 1997 and has not been heard from since. "Their mother wasn't well, possibly infected with HIV, and had returned to her village, which Zambians often do, to die," says Goodson Matenda, the 30-year-old Outreach manager.

Today with HIV/AIDS, every Zambian child is a potential street kid, says Matenda. "They are part and parcel of what this disease is doing to this country. We've found the children of church ministers, high government officials, lawyers, judges, living on the streets because their parents have died. Although not everyone is accepting of them, some give money. They now understand that but for the grace of God, their children could be on the streets, too."

While the general public may understand that, the government seems not to. In September 2000, Dawson Lupunga, Zambia's minister for community development and social services, announced he was launching a crackdown to arrest street kids. "If they're not being productive, they should leave the capital, find themselves land, and grow food on it," he said. It was a scathing, unrealistic, and unsympathetic response to the most devastating problem facing his country today.

As the government nods at the wheel, the welfare of Zambia's children is increasingly left to vastly underfunded nonprofit organizations, such as Fountain of Hope or Family Health Trust, one of the first nonprofit agencies to work against the spread of HIV/AIDS in the country. "The humanitarian agencies have contributed to the government's relaxation on AIDS. By doing their job for them, we've made them lazy," says the director of one foreign health agency.

Destruction of a Generation

A key area not being addressed is the psychological effect on children orphaned by this modern-day plague, says Elizabeth Mataka, Family Health Trust's executive director. "We need to understand the impact on youngsters watching their parents wither before their eyes and die, and then perhaps seeing their other siblings fall sick and die as well," Mataka says. "And just when the surviving children need the presence of those closest to them, they are split up and parceled out to different relatives, often living long distances away. The psychological impact of all this on children is very, very marked, and long term. If it is not addressed soon, we will end up with a country of very dysfunctional adults. People who are very angry at society are likely to be highly destructive."

The number of orphans is not expected to peak until 2030. "We underestimated the magnitude and urgency of the pandemic," says UNICEF's McDermott. But even United Nations (UN) epidemiologists, long experienced in charting the spread of such diseases, were surprised by the rapid growth of HIV in sub-Saharan Africa. In 1991, they underestimated the number of infections in the year 2000 by 40 percent. Already, 17 million have died, and in 2001 there are more than 25 million infected.

And so, Sundays in Zambia are punctuated by long funeral processions. As their childhoods end abruptly, legions of frightened and confused kids struggle to comprehend why their lives have so precipitously spun out of control. And their grandmothers, aunts, uncles, and older sisters work against all odds to support them.

Keeping Hope Alive

In the midst of what can sometimes appear to be insolvable AIDS-related troubles in Zambia, there are positive developments. Grassroots organizations, for example, are finding ways to support AIDS orphans—groups such as the one run by 65-year-old Elizabeth Ngoma in Matero, near Lusaka. Ngoma and other widowed grandmothers have banded together to support some 1200 orphans (some their own grandchildren) and pay school fees by selling scones. "We had to do something," says Ngoma. "We've become a village of grandmothers and orphans."

Some Zambian women are also beginning to cut their own risk of being infected by abstaining from sex. "In this culture of AIDS, I can only trust myself," says 26-year-old Eugenia Tembo. In the southwestern part of Zambia, kkiya, meaning "lockup," is quietly catching on among women who believe that when all other options are closed to men, they will stay faithful to their wives.

There is an increasing effort, too, to make men a part of the solution. Kondani Cephas Mwanza, 23, a counselor at Family Health Trust, is teaching young men about the plague. He has lost his parents, four brothers, and three sisters to AIDS. Mwanza himself was tested for HIV five years ago. "I was negative," he says, "and I haven't had sex since."

In the capital, in 2001 the HIV rate among pregnant 15- to 19-year olds is beginning to drop for the first time, thanks in part to the *Trendsetters* newspaper published by Cathy Phirl, 21, and her sister Mary, 24, who grew up in Sweden and returned to Lusaka with a more progressive approach to sex. With articles entitled "How to Tell Someone You Have HIV" and "Would You Die for Love?" *Trendsetters* has quickly won a loyal readership. "People ask us questions they can't ask their parents," says Cathy Phirl, "such as, 'Is it safer to use two condoms?' The answer is no, two are more likely to cause both to burst."

"We're big on abstinence," she says. "We do tell kids, however, that if they are sexually active, use a condom. It took a while but parents are now beginning to accept us. *Trendsetters* has also drawn attention from Johns Hopkins University in the U.S., which has helped with funding."

Phirl says it's important to realize that there is hope. "Twenty-five percent of our population is positive," she says, "but that means 75 percent is negative. Three out of four of us have the means to turn the situation around. But to do that, Zambians need to take control of their lives."

Preventing and Controlling Epidemics

Preparing for Epidemics in the United States

BY DAVID PERLIN AND ANN COHEN

David Perlin is the scientific director of the Public Health Research Institute, a nonprofit biomedical organization specializing in research on infectious diseases, that is part of the International Center for Public Health in Newark, New Jersey. He also lectures frequently on bioterrorism. Ann Cohen, now a full-time writer, was formerly the institute's director of public affairs. In this excerpt from The Complete Idiot's Guide to Dangerous Diseases and Epidemics, *Perlin and Cohen list the steps that they believe the United States should take to prevent future epidemics, whether natural or caused by terrorists. These steps include improvements in public health measures, communication between health agencies, and disease surveillance and diagnosis. Perlin and Cohen also explain how recent and expected advances in genetics may help physicians fight epidemics.*

Despite the optimism of the antibiotic era, infectious diseases are still a serious threat to us all. As political and technological advances continue to put people from all over the world in close contact with one another, the need for coordinated, international efforts to combat infectious diseases—especially those that are spread through the air—increases. Furthermore, the threat of bioterrorism is much more real after the events of fall 2001, and we need to do whatever we can to be prepared.

Our public health system must have the resources—financial, medical, and scientific—to rapidly identify the cause of an outbreak or epidemic and to treat victims appropriately. There must be coordination on all levels: local, state, federal, and international. Furthermore, public and private organizations must support cutting-edge research so that new technologies, drugs, diagnostics, and vaccines are discovered, developed, and made available quickly.

Improving Public Health Measures

For most of us, good public health programs are basically invisible. Our water is clean, safe, and drinkable. Garbage does not pile up on the streets. We vaccinate our children on a schedule suggested by the Centers for Disease Control and Prevention (CDC) and local health departments. Public health organizations track diseases such as rabies and tuberculosis without most people being aware of it.

In the fall of 2001, when anthrax was delivered through the mail to United States senators and television news stations, public health officials and organizations suddenly became more visible. Thousands looked to the CDC for guidance and answers. They wondered, "What do you do if you think you've been exposed to anthrax?" "Should you get your doctor to write a prescription for Cipro [an antibiotic used to treat anthrax]?" "Why did some people get Cipro and others get doxycyline [a different antibiotic]?" "Which drug is better and why?" "How rapidly can a potential anthrax exposure be confirmed?"

Despite conflicting opinions about how the anthrax cases were handled and how government agencies did or did not communicate with one another, there's no doubt that the public health system played an important role—without them, the outbreak might have been much worse. To be better prepared when the next attack or epidemic occurs, these organizations need better funding and support.

Communication

The United States has the most extensive disease surveillance and response network in the world. But there are gaps in its ability to detect outbreaks early.

In the case of West Nile virus in 1999, it took a long time to establish the link between dead birds and sick people. If there had been established communication links between those who deal with human health and those who deal with animal health, West Nile probably would have been identified much earlier.

When a new or unidentified disease appears, our public health system must be able to identify the disease, work across state, local, and federal lines to determine how widespread it is, and quickly implement an effective control plan.

First and foremost, this requires good communication. Turf issues and jurisdictions must take a back seat to finding out what is going on and containing it. Public health officials need to be willing to work across disciplines with physicians, researchers, and veterinarians.

Policies, planning, and training are needed to ensure that early detection and surveillance are effective. Even the most effective drugs and vaccines will be ineffective if we don't identify which ones we need. When policies are developed at the federal level, they must be shared with state and local officials so everyone is aware of them in case of disease outbreaks or bioterrorist attacks.

One of the most important things we need to do is to improve laboratories' capabilities. For example, only a few labs in the U.S. have the equipment and staff capable of performing diagnostic tests rapidly enough to deal with new and emerging diseases or bioterrorist attacks. We must upgrade our laboratories, taking advantage of new technologies that are being developed by top academic researchers around the world.

Surveillance

According to the World Health Organization (WHO), surveillance of infectious diseases is crucial for prevention and control. *Surveillance* is defined as the ongoing systematic collection, collation, analysis, and interpretation of data; and the dissemination of information to those who need to know so that action may be taken.

Surveillance is used to . . .

- Monitor disease trends.
- Monitor progress to see if methods used to control infections are working.
- Estimate the size of a health problem.
- Detect outbreaks of an infectious disease.
- Evaluate intervention and preventive programs.
- Identify research needs.

We can use the powerful computers now available to conduct disease surveillance programs and share data electronically. In 1992, scientists in New York and the Netherlands developed a database of "most-wanted" tuberculosis strains that were causing outbreaks in New York and elsewhere. A number of countries shared information about strains in their midst, and this gave those countries that were not experiencing outbreaks an opportunity to track their existing tuberculosis cases and identify a potential outbreak in its infancy. This began with the use of DNA fingerprinting technology to characterize different TB strains and a computer-matching program to compare the fingerprints.

The CDC developed a voluntary network that now includes more than 100 hospitals to share information on hospital infections. Unfortunately, with data from hospitals scattered throughout the country and reported infrequently, it is difficult to make judgments and develop policies regarding hospital infections. However, this type of program is a step in the right direction.

Certain diseases, such as tuberculosis, are reportable. In other words, any time a doctor or hospital finds a case, they are required

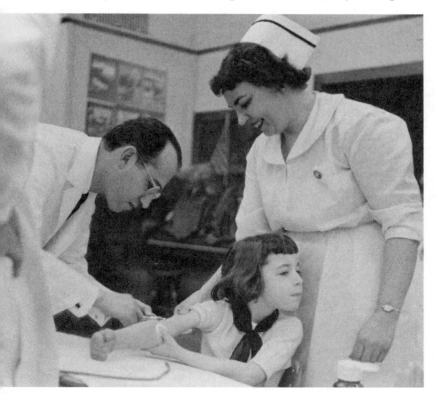

Research and the development of new vaccines helps the United States prevent future epidemics. Here, Dr. Jonas Salk, developer of the polio vaccine, vaccinates a child against the disease.

to contact their local or state health department. Reportability can be a tool for conducting effective surveillance.

Rapid Diagnosis

One of the most important elements of an effective public health program—one that can contain, control, and prevent disease—is the ability to rapidly identify the cause of an illness. Such identification involves determining the kind of organism causing the disease—is it a bacteria or a virus, for example—and whether it's susceptible or resistant to antibiotics. This information is crucial for figuring out how to treat sick patients, whether isolation is necessary, and who else around the patient should be tested for exposure to the disease.

Most diagnostic tests still depend on looking for the presence of antibodies—the immune system's response to attack by an external invader—in the blood. It usually takes between 24 and 48 hours to discern antibodies. In many cases, such tests are appropriate because the diseases aren't all that dangerous and early identification is not a life and death matter.

At times, though, speed is of the essence. Rapid identification of a resistant hospital infection, within hours, for example, could go a long way to both treating the patient and preventing the infection from spreading. Rapid identification of a tuberculosis infection, which can take weeks to diagnose, could help to slow the spread of this airborne organism.

Public health officials fear that future bioterrorist attacks could spread a genetically altered organism the likes of which we've never seen before. It could be a hybrid combination of a bacterium and a virus, or a bacterium genetically altered to produce a potent toxin from another bacterium. By using molecular techniques to diagnose an illness caused by such an organism, public health officials will be better able to identify the disease-causing organism, and thus take appropriate measures to stop the spread of the disease and treat people already infected with it.

To date, these new technologies have not been widely available to government and public health laboratories because they are in development and can be costly. It is important, however, that all the technologies and techniques that can be used to prevent the rapid spread of disease be made available to those who need them most, including public health and hospital laboratories. The days saved by not having to send a sample across the country for identification could save hundreds of lives.

One of the most important advances in molecular biology in recent years has been the sequencing of genomes of a number of organisms, as well as the sequencing of the human genome. Sequencing is the determination of the exact order of all the base pairs of DNA in an organism. Often specific genes are sequenced, too. How does this impact our approach to infectious diseases?

Medical researchers used to study an organism one gene at a time. With the availability of whole *genomes*, the entire genetic makeup of an organism, it's possible for researchers to study the whole organism as a system—looking at many or all of its genes at once. This method can help in the development of better preventive measures like vaccines, better diagnostics, and better treatments.

For example, the genomes [the microorganisms that cause infections] of some infectious diseases, such as staph[ylococcus] and tuberculosis, have already been sequenced. Researchers can determine how genes function in these organisms more quickly and, hopefully, find genes that are vital to the life of the organism—those are good targets for developing drugs that kill them.

Drug Development and the Human Genome

Researchers hope that [possessing the sequence of] the human genome will help them develop a new generation of drugs based on genes. Researchers will use gene sequence and function information to develop new drugs, instead of relying on the traditional [drug development methods] which basically involved trial and error. The drugs will be targeted to work at specific sites in the body, and should have fewer side effects than many of today's medicines.

The relatively new field of *pharmacogenomics* is the study of how a person's individual genetic makeup affects his or her body's response to drugs. It is possible that over time, drugs could be custom-made for individuals and adapted to each person's specific genetic makeup. Environment, diet, age, lifestyle, and state of health all can influence a person's response to medicines, but understanding a person's genetic makeup is thought to be the key to creating personalized drugs with greater safety and effectiveness.

Other potential benefits of pharmacogenomics include . . .

- **More powerful medicines** Drug companies and researchers may be able to develop drugs based on the actual proteins, enzymes, and RNA molecules associated with genes and diseases. This will allow them to produce medicines targeted to specific diseases. It is hoped that this accuracy will increase the drugs' effectiveness while decreasing damage to nearby healthy cells.

- **Better, safer drugs the first time** In time, doctors will be able to look at a patient's genetic profile and prescribe the best available therapy for that patient. This will help to lower the impact of side effects.
- **More accurate methods of determining appropriate dosages** Dosages today are based on the patient's weight and age. In the future, this will be replaced with dosages based on their genetic makeup. This will include how well the body processes the medicine and the time it takes to metabolize it. This will maximize the drug's effectiveness and decrease the likelihood of overdose.
- **Advanced screening for disease** Having your genetic makeup available will allow you to make appropriate lifestyle and environmental changes at an early age, to lessen the severity of a genetic disease. Knowing susceptibility in advance will also allow treatment to be used at the right time to maximize its effectiveness.
- **Better vaccines** Vaccines made of genetic material, either DNA or RNA, will provide all the benefits of existing vaccines with lower risk. They will activate the immune system but they won't cause infections. They will be inexpensive, stable, and easy to store.

Researchers and public health officials also hope that pharmacogenomics will help speed the approval process for new drugs. Clinical trials can be developed to target patients who are most likely to respond to a particular drug, reducing the risk of a part of a drug having catastrophic results.

If researchers can more quickly develop better drugs and determine what drugs will work most effectively on patients, it is possible that overall health-care costs will be reduced.

Gene Therapy

Gene therapy, or using people's own genes to treat disease, is still in the very early stages of development, but researchers are excited by its possibilities. It might be possible to use gene therapy to treat or even cure genetic and acquired diseases by using normal genes to replace or supplement a defective gene, or to bolster immunity to disease. For example, a gene could be modified to help stop tumor growth or to bolster immunity against certain disease-causing organisms.

Gene therapy is still in the experimental stages. Most experiments with it involve attempting to change a patient's genome to help them overcome a disease. This change would not be passed on to the next generation—the person's children—but there is early work being done on gene therapy that would target egg and sperm cells, with the goal of passing on the healthier genes to the next generation.

Basic Research

With all the excitement surrounding genomics and the new rapid molecular diagnostic methods, it's important to understand and appreciate the vital role that basic medical research plays in the advancement and improvement of health care around the world.

Researchers at private organizations, government agencies, pharmaceutical, and biotechnology companies figure out how microorganisms cause disease; find targets for drug, vaccine, and diagnostic development; and determine how disease-causing organisms become resistant to drugs. They study our body's immune responses and determine which of our genes are activated and how they work when we get sick.

The federal government provides significant support for researchers through the National Institutes of Health (NIH) and other agencies, including the Department of Defense. It is vital that this support continues to be a national priority and that new programs, such as bioterrorist-preparedness programs, include significant research components to help us stay a few steps ahead of the bugs.

The government must also encourage public-private collaborations and cooperation among research and academic organizations so that new advances are shared, to improve the health of people worldwide.

The bugs that cause disease have been around for 3.5 billion years. People have been around for a tiny fraction of that time, so the odds are the bugs will continue to evolve and outsmart our efforts to destroy them. We must be vigilant and continue to learn more about the bugs in order to figure out how we can co-exist with them so they don't destroy us.

Tracking Epidemics on the Internet

By Gary Taubes

In this article, award-winning science writer Gary Taubes, a frequent contributor to publications such as the New York Times, Science, Discover, *and* Technology Review*, describes several new infectious-disease surveillance systems that harness the power of the Internet. Taubes shows how these systems—ProMED-Mail, the Global Public Health Information Network (GPHIN), and Outbreak—help health care workers and researchers around the world keep in touch with each other and learn quickly about outbreaks in any part of the globe, a necessary first step in controlling the spread of epidemic diseases. He stresses that the systems' independence from governments and political agendas, as well as their use of the latest communications technology, helps them function effectively.*

The airplane brings disease home instantly. Epidemiologists are responding with electronic forms of quarantine. Despite its unsavory reputation as one of the legendary scourges of mankind, yellow fever is primarily a disease of animals—monkeys, in particular. In South America, the virus moves through the canopies of tropical rain forests in enormous waves. Carried by mosquitoes, its primary victims are howler monkeys, which are chimp-sized and notorious for being heard rather than seen. Researchers who study this jungle cycle of yellow fever say that they can tell when the waves of virus are rolling by because dead howlers start dropping out of trees. While the virus periodically finds its way into humans working

Gary Taubes, "Virus Hunting on the Web," *Technology Review*, vol. 101, November/December 1998. Copyright © 1998 by the Association of Alumni and Alumnae of MIT. Reproduced by permission.

in the rain forest, there hasn't been an urban epidemic in this hemisphere since 1942, a situation that has epidemiologists and public health experts holding their breath.

In their worst-case nightmares, a traveler or tourist contracts yellow fever in the Amazon, gets on a plane before symptoms appear and gets off 3,000 miles away, where he or she can be bitten by the local mosquitoes before the disease has been discovered or diagnosed, and the victim effectively quarantined. That such nightmares are not solely the stuff of imagination was demonstrated on the night of June 28, 1996, when a Swiss physician posted a case report on a Web site known as ProMED-Mail. The report was short and pithy: the story of a single unfortunate, unvaccinated tourist, who contracted yellow fever on a boat trip through the Amazon on April 5, and died 10 days later in a hospital in Basel. The fact that such episodes have not yet sparked a new wave of urban epidemics of yellow fever, according to New York State Health Department epidemiologist Jack Woodall, founder of ProMED-Mail, can be attributed to a single factor: "pure luck."

Helping News Catch Up with Disease

Welcome to the global village of emerging infectious pathogens, where the bubonic plague can erupt in India, Ebola in Zaire, or avian flu in Hong Kong, and any or all could make it to Boston in 12 hours; where a traveler returning home can spread a disease to his family, friends and co-workers before making it to the hospital, perhaps infecting everyone he comes into contact with.

To fight the threat—popularized in such books as Richard Preston's *The Hot Zone* and Laurie Garrett's *The Coming Plague*—epidemiologists and public health experts have been trying to come up with methods of monitoring diseases that match the electronic rapidity of modern times. Yet because many repressive governments are loath to publicize their health problems, the job of disease reporting has fallen to nongovernmental organizations, traditionally the World Health Organization (WHO). But the WHO will not release information on a potential epidemic until it has been reliably confirmed, which can take months. Public health experts who want their news now and not later have learned to rely on Woodall's ProMED-Mail.

ProMED-Mail (the name represents Program for Monitoring Emerging Diseases) is an Internet, e-mail based system connected by satellite to ground stations and Internet nodes throughout the world. It can be found at www.healthnet.org and anyone can subscribe. Fill in your e-mail address and a dozen postings a day will appear in your in-box—cholera in Pakistan, Rift Valley fever in Kenya, tick-borne encephalitis in Russia, E. coli infections in Wyoming. In the four years since it went online, ProMED-Mail has grown from 40 subscribers in seven countries to 15,000 in 150 and is now considered by experts to be an indispensable, although not wholly reliable, medium for transmitting news of outbreaks and connecting health experts to the far corners of the globe. Meanwhile, the WHO has joined with Health Canada to produce what they call the "Cadillac of ProMEDs," which was launched in early June 1998.

The ultimate goal of these electronic efforts is what Woodall calls "global transparency" of disease reporting. Ideally, within days of an outbreak, public health officials worldwide will know where and what has happened and be able to mobilize immediately, sending teams to help contain the outbreak at its source or warning local hospitals and ports of entry to watch for travelers who might have to be quarantined. While the Internet is assuredly the way to do it, says Duane Gubler, director of the division of vector-borne infectious diseases at the Centers for Disease Control and Prevention (CDC), no one is quite sure yet what form the ultimate monitoring system will take, or who will run it. "This is the wave of the future as far as disease surveillance is concerned," says Gubler. "Our challenge is how do we assure the quality of the reporting. If we can accomplish that and harness the thing properly, it's going to be the best thing that ever happened to disease surveillance."

An Experienced Epidemiologist

To initiate a surveillance network that intends to cover the entire world, not to mention the entire spectrum of infectious disease epidemiology, it helps to have wide experience in the field, which is definitely the case with Woodall. He was raised in China by English parents and schooled in mosquito-borne diseases at the London School of Hygiene and Tropical Medicine. He has worked on yellow fever in Uganda and hemorrhagic fever in Bolivia, done lab work in the old Rockefeller Foundation labs in Manhattan and at Yale University in New Haven, and has run virus labs in the Amazon rain forest and in Puerto Rico. Before moving to Albany to take up his post with the New York State Health Department, he spent 13 years as an international health expert working for the WHO in Geneva. "Although I wasn't just in Geneva," he says. "I traveled all over the world—China, Africa, all over. Because I was the only virologist in Geneva who spoke Portuguese, I ended up setting up the first AIDS programs in the Portuguese-speaking countries of Africa. I did all kinds of things. I was a jack-of-all-trades."

Woodall eventually ended up in the WHO branch of epidemiology, surveillance and health statistics, which is where he was when he started down the path that led to ProMED-Mail. After co-authoring a paper on biological weapons disarmament, as Woodall tells it, he ended up on the Iraq desk of the WHO during the Gulf War [in 1991]. In 1993, that assignment brought him into contact with the Federation of American Scientists, which was co-sponsoring a meeting in Geneva with the WHO on a program to set up ProMED centers around the world that could monitor outbreaks of emerging pathogens as well as the kind of disease activity that might signify biological warfare and bioterrorist activities. Woodall was in charge of the task force on communication, whose goal was to determine how best to connect the centers.

Satellites Meet the Internet

While the centers have yet to be funded, Woodall took his part of the project and developed it into ProMED-Mail, with the crucial help of SatelLife, a Boston-based organization founded in 1989 by Bernard Lown. Lown is a cardiologist and inventor—of the defibrillator [a device that uses electric current to control rapid, abnormal heartbeats] most famously—and founder of the International Physicians for the Prevention of Nuclear War, an association that won the Nobel Peace Prize in 1985. After winning the prize, Lown set out to establish a network that would bridge the gap between medicine in the developed and underdeveloped worlds.

Lown decided that the technology needed to accomplish that task was a communications satellite dedicated to the purpose. In 1989, SatelLife became the first nonprofit organization in the world to launch its own communications satellite, HealthSat 1, which was supplanted in 1993 by HealthSat 2. The satellite, roughly the size of a television set, circles the globe every 100 minutes in a "low-Earth" orbit at an altitude of 550 miles. It passes over ground stations anywhere from four to 14 times a day, at which times the ground stations can upload or download messages. When the satellite is over Boston it downloads incoming messages to the SatelLife offices and takes on outgoing mail. The ground stations themselves are simple: desktop computers with a small radio and an omnidirectional antenna. "Uploading and downloading e-mail four times a day doesn't sound like much today," says Woodall, "but even today in countries like Zaire with no telephone and no e-mail provider, four times a day is a hell of a lot better than nothing at all."

In 1994 Woodall was introduced to SatelLife executives, who offered to host ProMED-Mail for free until funding could be obtained. ProMED-Mail officially went online that August with a $50,000 startup grant from the Rockefeller Foundation, $1,000 a month for expenses from the Federation of American Sciences, and SatelLife subsidizing the rest. Woodall enlisted half a dozen chronically overworked and unpaid moderators to serve as editors and to oversee the correspondence and weed out the more obvious rumor-mongering.

The "CNN of Outbreaks"

After four years, Woodall calls ProMED-mail the "CNN of outbreaks," a description few epidemiologists dispute. "We have more subscribers from the CDC alone then we have from any other entire country in the world except Australia," says Woodall. "We have subscribers from NIH [National Institutes of Health], FDA [the Food and Drug Administration], you name it; they know we're the place to get breaking news on outbreaks."

ProMED has proven over the years that if an epidemic breaks out anywhere in the world, you're likely to hear about it first there, from dengue in Malaysia to a 1996 Ebola outbreak in Gabon. If the information does not come from government health agencies, it is likely to come from a physician or missionary working in the middle of nowhere, which was the case with the Gabon Ebola outbreak. "We had information from the Central African Republic before anybody else had it," says Charlie Callisher, a ProMED moderator at Colorado State University. "Not that we go out necessarily looking for it, but there are missionaries out there who read ProMED. They're thrilled they have it. It keeps them in touch with the outside world, and if they see something funny, they tell us first."

The story of the Swiss tourist who succumbed to yellow fever is a classic case of ProMED's impact. The Swiss physician who reported the case got to ProMED only after Woodall noticed a submission the doctor had made to a Web site known as Outbreak, for which Woodall serves as chief of the scientific review team. When the physician mentioned he had seen a case of yellow fever, Woodall promptly asked him to post a case report on ProMED, which led to the WHO and Pan American Health Organizations (PAHO) learning of the situation. PAHO informed the Brazilian government, which initiated a vaccination campaign in Manaus to avoid a possible outbreak. "It's a damn good thing they did," says Woodall. "Six months later the same thing happened to an American tourist. He had been told to get vaccinated, but couldn't be bothered. He went to the same area, went fishing on the Amazon, got sick, went through Manaus, waited overnight for a plane, and got back to Tennessee to die."

Worldwide Expertise

So far the most impressive aspect of ProMED has been its ability to channel expertise to those who desperately need it. Since virtually everyone in the epidemiological world follows ProMED, a request for advice or expertise will get immediate response, sometimes from the single best source. This was vividly illustrated in March 1997, when a researcher with the National Institute for Virology in Johannesburg, South Africa, posted a message about plans by the South African government to build low-cost housing on the site of a medical hospital cemetery where smallpox victims had been buried as late as 1950. The researcher worried whether there was a risk of the smallpox virus remaining viable [alive and able to cause disease] over all this time. "Smallpox immunization is unavailable," he wrote, "and if viable smallpox is released into the nonimmune population of Johannesburg, we have a disaster on our hands."

To answer the query, Callisher went to Frank Fenner of the Australian National University, who was chair of the WHO committee overseeing the final demise of the smallpox virus. He posted Fenner's response explaining that the risk of smallpox still being around after 40 years was "vanishingly small" and that bones would not harbor live virus in any case. Callisher also advised the South Africans to contact another world authority on smallpox who happened to live in Capetown and provided the phone number.

Independence from Governments

One of the advantages of a system such as ProMED-Mail is that it has no governmental affiliation, and so it can freely ignore the desire of some governments to cover up their health problems. This is why Woodall and his colleagues say a CDC-run monitoring system, for instance, is sure to be inadequate. "Because we're independent," says Woodall, "we don't need anybody's permission other than the author's to put anything out." Or as Callisher says, "We have to have a free exchange of information. A government ProMED wouldn't work."

The ultimate example came in 1997 when a dengue epidemic hit Cuba after the Cuban government had been claiming since the early 1980s that the mosquito vector for dengue had been eradicated. As the dengue epidemic spread, the Cuban government reported several thousand cases and 10 to 20 deaths. These numbers differed dramatically from those put out by an independent news agency known as CubaPress, which was picked up by ProMED. CubaPress was getting its numbers from Dr. Desi Mendoza, the founder of the Independent Medical College of Santiago de Cuba, who was arrested by Cuban police for disseminating information on the epidemic to foreign journalists. The arrest was played out in ProMED along with the epidemic and the ongoing attempts to pressure the Cubans to free Mendoza. ProMED kept reporting on the Cuban situation as long as CubaPress was in business. When the independent news agency stopped sending out information, ProMED lost touch.

The Risk of Rumors

The fact that ProMED provides such rapid access is a great strength; yet that same rapidity of access can breed problems with quality control—they're the flip side of the coin in the electronic age. Callisher and his monitors are overworked and underfunded, and they can't fact-check every entry that comes their way. This unavoidable situation led to criticism that ProMED-Mail disseminates rumors. Gubler, for instance, says that if he allowed himself to do so, he could spend entirely too much of his time correcting ProMED misinformation. David Heymann, who directs the WHO's Division of Emerging and Other Communicable Diseases (EMC), calls ProMED a "very valuable service," but adds that the WHO does not participate in their discussions, because the organization is "not in a position to discuss rumors with the general public." The WHO goal, he says, is to get the rumors and check them out.

After the 1995 Ebola outbreak in Zaire, the WHO established Heymann's EMC, which oversees the organization's global surveillance networks. The network collects information from some 1,000 laboratory centers around the world, including more than 200 specializing in infectious diseases. "For arboviruses [arthropod-borne viruses, usually carried by insects] and hemorrhagic fevers," explains Heymann, "we have 37 labs throughout the world constantly receiving specimens to look for Ebola, dengue, and yellow fever. The results are given to WHO and to the country where the specimen originates. We then look to validate the results, and if it's an outbreak situation, we look to get the necessary groups involved, to make sure the outbreak is addressed and contained."

The WHO says it receives as many as five unconfirmed rumors a week of new infectious-disease outbreaks, by telephone, newspaper or e-mail. Each rumor is then investigated and a rumor/ outbreak list is sent out electronically on a need-to-know basis to relevant personnel at the WHO, its collaborating centers and other public health authorities. These reports, however, are not intended for public consumption. The WHO will only post news of an outbreak on the EMC's public Web page after confirmation. Because confirmation often requires sending specimens to a laboratory that may be outside the country of origin, the WHO system is notoriously slow at alerting the world at large to outbreaks.

An Expanded System

To strengthen the system and accelerate its response time, the WHO has recently joined with Health Canada to create the Global Public Health Information Network (GPHIN), which Heymann says will "really be the system" because it will subsume ProMED within it. GPHIN will include all the reports from ProMED, but also will incorporate information gathered from other sources.

GPHIN is the brainchild of Rudi Nowak, a Canadian physician and public health specialist and former director of Canadian quarantine operations. Nowak says that he realized the contemporary world had drastically changed the nature of his business and that the problem had to be addressed. "We're not talking quarantine the way it used to be," he says. "People boarded a ship in Europe, for instance, and it took them 11 or 12 days to come to North America, and some got sick and died, and those that were sick were put into quarantine when they arrived. Now people can get anywhere within hours, and they can get exposed to serious pathogens without even knowing it and get back home within the incubation period of the disease." The way Nowak likes to put it is that quarantine has moved "from the seaport to the emergency room."

GPHIN uses a search engine to scan the Web continuously for all information pertaining to infectious diseases, including specific sites such as ProMED. The search engine stores the findings under six headings: cholera, salmonella, hemorrhagic fevers, antibiotic resistance, encephalitis, and floods. The latter, says Nowak, "because if you have floods, cholera is just around the corner."

GPHIN then further breaks the incoming information into three bins, depending on how urgently they have to be addressed: a "hot" bin, for the first report of outbreaks; a "standby" bin, for collateral information on existing situations; and a bin for rejected information, which can include worthless rumors and irrelevant information. GPHIN then extracts the relevant information from each report and places it in an "intelligence" report that can be scanned quickly. This step is currently carried out by humans, says Nowak, but only until commercial artificial intelligence technology is available.

When users enter the Web site, they'll start with the latest intelligence reports, and if they want more detailed information they can go to the original reports from which the intelligence was gathered. "Initially they can simply come in and say, 'Let's look at the cholera bin and see what's happened around the world in the last 24 hours.' They can then scan through reports as they come in." GPHIN is also fully interactive and so, as with ProMED, anyone reading the page who has something important to add can do so.

Nowak and his collaborators officially launched GPHIN in early June, and the system began searching the Web in both French and English. Eventually, it will expand to all seven WHO official languages. What the system won't do—unlike ProMED— is report to the public. The current system is designed for public health officials and no one else. "We cannot really be accused of being in the business of spreading rumors," says Nowak. "The information sooner or later will be available to the general public, but it has to be verified. We don't want to create unnecessary anxiety among the public."

With a little luck, ProMED and GPHIN will both take care of what CDC arbovirus researcher Paul Reiter suggests has been the regrettable history of infectious disease fighting to date. To put it simply, he says, all the monitoring and surveillance has only served to mobilize the world's resources to fight "ex-epidemics. Whenever we've been sent out to epidemics, we've always arrived when the epidemic was pretty much history." He cites, for example, a 1993 yellow fever epidemic in Kenya, at which the medical cavalry arrived in time to see the last two cases. Or, going way back, a yellow fever epidemic in the Omo River Valley in Ethiopia between 1960 and 1962. "You had something like a million people susceptible to yellow fever," says Reiter, "with 30,000 deaths"; no one outside Ethiopia, he says, "had the faintest idea until it was all over." Now with the Internet the news should get out in time to make a difference. "We're primed," he says.

A Strategy for Global Infectious Disease Surveillance

BY THE WORLD HEALTH ORGANIZATION

Founded in 1948 by the United Nations, the World Health Organization (WHO) combats epidemics worldwide and advises countries on developing health services and improving the health of their citizens. WHO describes its strategy for spotting and tracking epidemics in this 1998 fact sheet. The organization explains its role in global disease surveillance and lists the formal, informal, and legally mandated sources of information on which it relies. It presents its influenza surveillance system as an example of its surveillance and monitoring programs and briefly describes what it will do when an outbreak or epidemic is detected.

Increased movements of people, expansion of international trade in foodstuffs and medicinal biological products, social and environmental changes linked to urbanization, and deforestation are all manifestations of the rapidly changing nature of the world we live in. Add to that the rapid adaptation of microorganisms, which has facilitated the return of old communicable diseases and the emergence of new ones, and the evolution of antimicrobial resistance, which means that curative treatments for a wide range of parasitic, bacterial and viral infections have become less effective, and a communicable disease in one country today is the concern of all.

During 1996, fatal yellow fever infections were imported into the United States and Switzerland by tourists who travelled to

yellow fever endemic areas without having had yellow fever vaccination. During the same year approximately 10,000 reported
cases of malaria were imported into the European Community,
with one fourth of them reported from the United Kingdom.
When cholera re-entered Peru in 1991, after a long absence, it
found an opportunity to spread through the existing sanitation
and water systems, causing over 3,000 deaths. Seafood exports
were embargoed from Peru and tourism decreased, costing an estimated loss of at least US$770 million to the Peruvian economy
in one year.

In industrialized countries where communicable disease mortality has greatly decreased over the past century, the concern is
preventing diseases from entering and causing an outbreak or reemergence. In developing countries, the concern is detecting
communicable disease outbreaks early and stopping their mortality, spread and potential impact on trade and tourism.

One of the major means of addressing the concerns about
communicable diseases in both industrialized and developing
countries is through the development of strong surveillance systems. However, in view of the disparity among national surveillance systems, partnerships in global surveillance are a logical
starting point in this area of common commitment.

WHO's Role in Disease Surveillance

Since 1992, alarm over emerging and re-emerging diseases has
resulted in a number of national and international initiatives to
restore and improve surveillance and control of communicable
diseases. The Member States of the World Health Organization
(WHO) expressed their concern in a resolution of the World
Health Assembly in 1995, urging all Member States to strengthen
surveillance for infectious diseases in order to promptly detect re-
emerging diseases and identify new infectious diseases. The World
Health Assembly recognized that the success of this resolution
depends on the ability to obtain information on infectious diseases and the willingness to communicate this information na-
tionally and internationally. Improved detection and surveillance,
moreover, will lead to better prioritizing of public health efforts.

One of WHO's main means of creating a global surveillance
system has been the development of a "network of networks"
which links together existing local, regional, national and international networks of laboratories and medical centres into a su-

per surveillance network. This network is being constructed together with the 191 WHO Member States and other partners, including the European Union–United States Task Force on Emerging Communicable Diseases and the US–Japan Common Agenda; the network has also been cited as an area of collaboration by the G-7/G-8 member countries at both the Lyon (1996) and the Denver (1997) Summit Meetings. Requirements for monitoring the intentional use of pathogenic microbes have also been addressed by the network, specifically in the revision of the International Health Regulations (IHR), and in collaboration with the ad hoc Group of States Parties to the Biological Weapons Convention.

Formal Sources of Information

Government and university centres of excellence in communicable diseases such as the US Centers for Disease Control and Prevention, the UK Public Health Laboratory Service, the French Pasteur Institutes, the global network of schools of public health and the Training in Epidemiology and Public Health Intention Network (TEPHINET) provide confirmed reports of communicable diseases. Most of these sites are or will become part of the WHO Collaborating Centre network. This network, along with the WHO Regional Offices, WHO country representatives and other WHO and UNAIDS, [the Joint United Nations Programme on HIV/AIDS] reporting sites, contributes to global surveillance along with reporting networks of other United Nations agencies such as UNHCR [Office of the United Nations High Commissioner for Refugees] and UNICEF [United Nations International Children's Emergency Fund, now United Nations Children's Fund]. International military networks such as the US Department of Defense Global Emerging Infections System (DoD-GEIS), private clinics, individual scientists and public health practitioners complete the network of formal information sources.

There are geographic and population gaps, as well as deficiencies in expertise in these networks, which must be rectified. As most of these networks represent the public sector, they should develop means of including the private sector, as well as other sources of valid information such as military and research laboratories. They need to represent both human and animal infections and provide information on antimicrobial resistance and the environment including water, insect vectors and animal reservoirs.

Informal Sources of Information

The rapid global reach in telecommunications, media and Internet access has created an information society permitting public health professionals to communicate more effectively. Many groups, including health professionals, nongovernmental organizations and the general public, now have access to reports on disease outbreaks, challenging national disease surveillance authorities which were once the sole source of such information. Public Internet sites are dedicated to disease news and include medicine and biology-related sites as well as those of the major news agencies and wire services. ProMed, an early electronic discussion site on communicable diseases occurrence on the Internet, provides an example.

Electronic discussion sites, accessible through free and unrestricted subscription, are valuable sources of information. Their scope may be worldwide (ProMed, TravelMed), regional (PACNET in the Pacific region) or national (Sentiweb in France). They exemplify unprecedented potential for increasing public awareness on public health issues.

The Global Public Health Information Network (GPHIN) is a second generation electronic surveillance system developed and maintained by Health Canada. It has powerful search engines that actively trawl the World Wide Web looking for reports of communicable diseases and communicable disease syndromes in electronic discussion groups, on news wires and elsewhere on the Web. GPHIN has begun to search in English and French and will eventually expand to all official languages of the World Health Organization, to which it has created close links for verification.

Other networks which are likewise sources for communicable disease reporting include nongovernmental organizations such as the Red Cross and Red Crescent Societies, Medecins sans Frontières [Doctors Without Borders], Medical Emergency Relief International (Merlin), and Christian religious organizations such as the Catholic and Protestant mission networks.

Legally Mandated Sources of Information

The International Health Regulations (IHR) are a legal instrument which requires WHO Member States to notify [inform authorities about cases of] diseases of international importance: currently plague, cholera and yellow fever. Countries have not uniformly complied with disease notification, often fearing unwarranted reactions that affect travel and trade. In addition, the official international reporting mechanism has not evolved with the new communications environment, and does not include many communicable diseases of importance to international public health. A revision of the IHR is therefore being directed towards a stronger role in global communicable disease surveillance and control. The revised IHR emphasize the immediate notification of all disease outbreaks of urgent international importance. This concept is currently being evaluated in a pilot study in 21 countries. Electronic reporting of specific clinical syndromes, which were developed taking into account those diseases of importance to public health, will help countries report immediately. This will facilitate rapid alert and appropriate international response while awaiting laboratory verification. Once the confirmed diagnosis is known it will also feed into the system, permitting any adjustments to the international response which may be necessary. When the revision is complete, the IHR will constitute an important public health tool.

A Practical Example: Global Influenza Surveillance

Influenza surveillance is one of the most developed global surveillance and monitoring systems of WHO. It started in 1948 and has developed over the years into a highly successful global partnership. In 1998, the network involves 110 collaborating laboratories in 82 countries, constantly monitoring locally isolated influenza viruses and providing information on true emergence and spread of different strains.

National case detection systems and laboratories have been strengthened by WHO and its partners using internationally accepted norms, and virus isolates from the national laboratories are analysed in more detail in one of the four WHO Collaborating Centres for Influenza. The data are then used by experts associated with the surveillance system to make recommendations on the three virus strains to be included in the next season's influenza vaccine. Thus, information generated from global surveillance results in an important and unified public health response each year. The annual design of the vaccine also represents an outstandingly successful collaboration between the public and private sectors.

In parallel to the surveillance programme, national and global pandemic plans are being developed to systematically address the next influenza pandemic. Both the surveillance system and the elements of the global pandemic plan were tested during the outbreak of the avian influenza A(H5N1) virus in human subjects in Hong Kong in late 1997. The rapid identification of the virus strain in one of the collaborating laboratories in the Netherlands, followed by the mobilization and coordination of an investigating team from WHO Collaborating Centres in the United States, extensive epidemiological and laboratory studies, the prompt dissemination of public information, the development of diagnostic test kits for international distribution, and the identification of a virus line suitable for vaccine development all contributed to a timely, ordered and effective response to the outbreak.

WHO's Epidemic Preparedness and Response

Once a communicable disease outbreak has been confirmed, pertinent information is placed on the World Wide Web and can be accessed by the general public (http://www.who.ch/emc/ outbreak_news/). At the same time, an international response, with the input of technical and humanitarian partners, is mounted if required. A WHO team arrives on site within 24 hours of outbreak confirmation to make an initial assessment and begin immediate control measures and prepare the ground for the larger international response if needed. By linking the international response to systematic global surveillance, a worldwide "network of networks" is available from which to solicit support, thus ensuring that no one country, technical or humanitarian partner must bear the entire burden.

The Plan to Fight Smallpox

By Geoffrey Cowley

Smallpox was eradicated worldwide in the late 1970s, but stocks of the smallpox (variola) virus still exist and, as Newsweek *health and medicine editor Geoffrey Cowley explains, many fear that bioterrorists might use them to start a new epidemic of the deadly disease. Because Americans have not been vaccinated against smallpox for decades, most people have little or no immunity to the disease, Cowley says. He presents a new government plan to deal with this threat, which includes increasing stockpiles of smallpox vaccine and preparing to vaccinate the country's entire population if necessary. He states, however, that government officials and health care experts still disagree about whether vaccination should be given preventatively or administered only after an epidemic has begun. Cowley's articles, on subjects ranging from AIDS to heart attack risk factors and dietary supplements, have won numerous awards.*

Smallpox is a ghost to most modern doctors—the greatest killer in history, perhaps, but not the sort of problem that shows up in one's waiting room. Dr. Donald Millar and Dr. Michael Lane are old enough to share a different perspective. Both took part in the U.S. government's smallpox-eradication efforts in the heady days of the 1960s and '70s. While chasing the variola [smallpox] virus through Africa and India, they saw what smallpox can do. The disease engulfs the body in pustules that itch and ooze, and often blind or disfigure victims lucky enough to survive. They also witnessed the power of a relatively crude vaccine to contain the awful killer. Both men believed deeply in the ideal of global eradication, but by 1969 they'd grown skeptical of the need for routine vaccination in the United States. American kids were no longer threatened by

smallpox, they wrote in *The New England Journal of Medicine*—
yet 7 million were still getting shots each year, thousands were
suffering adverse reactions and roughly 1 in a million was dying
of complications.

"The benefits of routine . . . vaccination no longer outweigh
its risks," the virus hunters concluded in a seminal phrase, "and
consideration should be given to its discontinuance."

A Virus Very Much Alive

Millar and Lane got their wish. The United States abandoned
routine smallpox vaccination in 1972, and never regretted the de-
cision. No one on earth has contracted natural smallpox since
1977. The World Health Organization declared the disease "eradicated" in 1980, and no country has vaccinated children since
1984. Unfortunately the variola virus, which causes smallpox, is
still very much alive. The Soviet government cultivated a huge
stockpile for military use during the 1980s, in violation of international law. The stockpile was eventually destroyed, and today
the only acknowledged variola samples are held in government
laboratories in the United States and Russia. But the Soviet
stockpile has never been fully accounted for. And events in 2001
and 2002—the World Trade Center attack, the anthrax attacks,
the persistence of Al Qaeda and the mounting hostilities with
Saddam Hussein—have lent new urgency to an old question.
Could terrorists hit us with smallpox?

The odds are impossible to gauge, but there is no question
we're vulnerable. Even as they called for an end to routine vaccination, Millar and Lane warned that the loss of widespread immunity would "raise our susceptibility to smallpox as a weapon
of biologic warfare." Those of us vaccinated before 1972 may still
have some residual protection, but the 119 million Americans
born since then are about as defenseless as the ones who greeted
Columbus 500 years ago. "Although smallpox has long been
feared as the most devastating of all infectious diseases," the Johns
Hopkins–based Working Group on Civilian Biodefense has written, "its potential for devastation today is far greater than at any
previous time."

Mass Vaccinations

Federal officials are as concerned as anyone else, and the Bush
administration has made "biosecurity" a high priority. At the

start of October 2002 the federal government came forward with a blueprint for quickly vaccinating the whole country in the event of a smallpox attack. And Health and Human Services [HHS] Secretary Tommy Thompson has presented the White House with a plan that could lead to routine "pre-attack" vaccination of up to 10 million health and emergency workers—and perhaps even private citizens—by early 2004. The HHS plan doesn't have a precise timetable, but it includes three phases. To start, the government would vaccinate the 500,000 health workers most likely to encounter patients during an outbreak. Later, as new vaccine stocks are developed and licensed by the Food and Drug Administration, other emergency workers would become eligible. And once that has happened, private citizens would gain voluntary access. In mid-October the proposal is not yet policy, just an option that the president will mull as he contemplates his next move in the "war on terror." Around October 7, members of the team that crafted it spoke at length to *Newsweek* about its origins and evolution, and the prospects for keeping America safe from smallpox. Their mood was summed up by Tom Ridge, director of the Office of Homeland Security. "You have people in this world who hate America and who have said they will use any means to harm us," he said, "You have to be prepared."

If embraced by the White House, the new plan will mark a sharp departure from the smallpox policies of the past three decades. When federal health officials abandoned routine vaccination in 1972, they assumed that "ring vaccination" would be an adequate substitute. The ring strategy involves isolating anyone with a suspected case of the pox, and quickly vaccinating the person's "primary contacts" (friends, family and co-workers) and "secondary contacts" (contacts of the contacts) in an expanding circle. The strategy is an efficient way to contain natural outbreaks. But as Yale health analyst Edward Kaplan observes, "It's a fantasy to believe that the control of small natural outbreaks provides guidance for large bioterrorist attacks." Anyone with the means and motivation to spread smallpox would presumably target a transportation hub or an urban crossroad, not a country store. By the time the first victims developed malaise [feelings of tiredness and weakness], fever and rash a week later, others infected at the same time could be dispersed throughout the country.

At the urging of the federal Centers for Disease Control and Prevention, state and local governments are now devising plans to vaccinate *everyone* during a smallpox attack. Health workers would still track and vaccinate the contacts of known victims. But under the new plan, laid out in a 48-page "Smallpox Vaccination Clinic Guide," states and cities must also establish clinics that can open quickly during an emergency to screen, counsel and vaccinate anyone who walks through the door. The CDC guide includes blueprints for model clinics in which staffs of 117 workers can vaccinate nearly 3,000 people during each eight-hour shift. Most experts agree that if health departments can pull off what the Feds have in mind, the mass-vaccination strategy will save lives. Smallpox doesn't spread easily from person to person during its seven- to 17-day incubation period, and even infected people can often avoid serious illness if they're vaccinated within four days. Inoculating the nation that quickly would pose enormous challenges, says Kaplan, "but it's not impossible at all."

New Vaccine Stockpiles

He couldn't have said that in 2001. When Ridge founded the Homeland Security Office in the Fall of that year, smoke was rising from Ground Zero, anthrax was moving through the nation's mail system and an exercise called "Dark Winter" had shown that, in Ridge's words, "we didn't have enough smallpox vaccine to inoculate the public on short notice." The government's entire inventory consisted of 15.4 million doses of Dryvax, a vaccine that Wyeth-Ayerst Laboratories made in the 1970s by injecting calves with vaccinia (a milder cousin of the variola virus) and harvesting more of it from the resulting blisters. Today, thanks to a series of lucky breaks, the Feds are sitting on more than a half-billion doses. The first break came when researchers discovered that the government's Dryvax was potent enough to use at one fifth the intended concentration. Suddenly, 15.4 million doses became 77 million. Then Thompson confirmed that Aventis Pasteur had come up with 86 million doses (which could be stretched to 430 million) of a virtually identical vaccine dating back to the 1950s. Aventis had been meaning to dispose of the stuff, says company spokesman Len Lavenda, but hadn't gotten around to it. So the firm converted the freeze-dried bulk into clinic-ready vaccine and handed it off to the government.

While stockpiling the old vaccines for emergencies, the government has also ordered up 210 million doses of a second-generation vaccine grown in cell cultures rather than cow pustules. That vaccine, developed by Acambis of Cambridge, England, will contain the same virus as the older ones and carry most of the same risks, but it will be less likely to harbor impurities. HHS expects to have 70 million doses on hand by the end

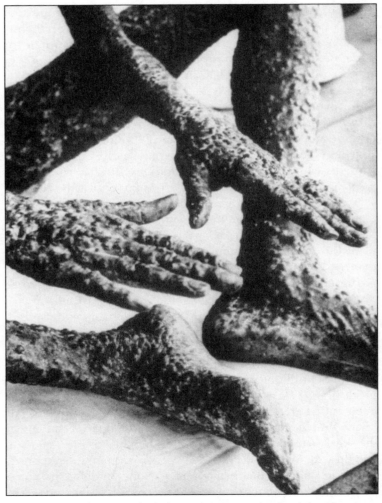

The smallpox virus causes the body to erupt in pustules that itch and ooze. Survivors of the disease often end up blind or disfigured.

of 2002. Meanwhile, no one is sweating over a shortage of vaccine. "In an emergency," says Dr. Anthony Fauci of the National Institute of Allergy and Infectious Diseases, "we'd have enough to vaccinate everybody tomorrow."

Racing to Be Ready

Local health officials are aghast at all the new chores they've inherited, but most profess confidence that they'll have disaster plans ready by Dec. 1, 2002, as the Feds have requested. New York City has a head start. "Fall 2001 was overwhelming," says Marci Layton, the city's assistant commissioner for communicable-disease control, "and that was just eight cases of anthrax. At the time, I said, 'Can you imagine what it would be like to respond to smallpox?'" The city has since expanded its monitoring system to pick up unusual patterns of infection throughout the five boroughs. Dr. Laurene Mascola may face even greater challenges as communicable-disease chief for Los Angeles County. Like Layton, she serves nearly 10 million constituents who speak dozens of languages. But her community is spread over 4,000 square miles. "You know that the first day a case is announced they're all going to knock on some door saying, 'Where's my vaccine?'" Mascola says. Her department has already developed a 153-page document with vaccination plans for outbreaks ranging from fewer than 10 cases to more than 1,000.

Big-city health departments aren't the only ones racing to be ready. In Butler County, Pa., Dr. Mark Carlsson is turning the fall 2002 flu-vaccine drive into a dry run for a smallpox campaign. Health workers will practice triaging patients and getting informed consent—and patients will report risk factors ranging from eczema [a skin disease] to AIDS to keep the workers on their toes. In Illinois, meanwhile, health workers are learning to prick orange skins with the once common bifurcated [split] needles that are used to jab vaccinia into people's upper arms. "Each time you go in, you put a little bit of that vaccine under the skin," state health director John Lumpkin explains, "and you end up with a mild infection that triggers an immune response." Lumpkin launched the smallpox-preparedness program in winter 2001–2002 and hopes to have 1,000 health workers trained by spring 2003.

Being prepared surely beats the alternative. But emergencies have a way of defying carefully laid plans. Just think back to 2001's anthrax scare, says Neal Cohen, a former New York City health commissioner who now heads a preparedness group called the Center on Bioterrorism. Experts predicted confidently that postal workers wouldn't be infected by sealed mail—until they were. And they dismissed the possibility that one tainted letter could contaminate others—until it happened. "A lot of our assumptions turned out to be faulty," he says. "We learned how little we really understood about the risks." Could freeway traffic stall response plans in L.A. or Atlanta? What about airport closures? And suppose terrorists managed to combine a small-pox release with a September 11–style assault that placed competing demands on the response system? "If there's more than one form of attack," says Millar, the virus hunter, "the task of vaccinating everyone in the country in a week becomes mind-boggling."

Competing Strategies

This is where the debate over preparedness gets interesting. Millar and Lane, the coauthors of that 1969 challenge to routine vaccination, remain fond friends 33 years later. But they have come to different conclusions about how best to prepare ourselves. Lane believes a post-attack strategy is the only one we need, but Millar favors voluntary peacetime vaccination as a strategy for restoring some of our lost immunity. The approach offers some indisputable advantages. For one thing, it could minimize the damage done by the vaccine itself. According to the CDC's latest estimates, 15 of every million first-time vaccinees could suffer life-threatening reactions to the vaccine—conditions such as encephalitis (brain inflammation), generalized vaccinia (a systemic infection from the vaccinia virus) and eczema vaccinatum (a widespread skin eruption). During peacetime, clinics could be more rigorous about taking people's medical histories and screening them for risk factors such as allergies, pregnancy or compromised immunity—which is far more common today than 30 years ago. And people who did react badly to the vaccine would stand a better chance of getting adequate care and medication. If even half the population were vaccinated in advance, everyone would be safer because fewer people would be capable of spreading the infection. And that in itself would make the variola virus a less attractive weapon. "We have proven preventive measures," says Dr. Bill Bicknell of Boston University's School of Public Health. "We've just spent millions on airport security. We could spend less on smallpox and just take it off the table."

Here's the catch, though. We *know* that smallpox vaccines cause harm. That's why we shelved them 30 years ago. Smallpox, however scary, is only a theoretical threat, and many experts insist it's an unlikely one—if only because the risk of "blowback" is so high. In an age of constant travel and low immunity, a large epidemic in any part of the world could quickly spread to others. Lane notes that Iraq hasn't vaccinated its people in decades and would have a hard time doing so today. "If [Saddam] is at all rational," he says, "then he knows that the more successful the attack, the more dangerous smallpox will be to him and other countries in the region." Presumably even suicide bombers and Al Qaeda's vandals, with their dreams of glorious martyrdom, don't want to destroy their own cultures. True, a peacetime vaccination effort could save us from a sophisticated nihilist who cares not who he kills. But if we're that averse to risk, why worry only about smallpox? Should we launch campaigns to vaccinate ourselves against the Marburg virus? asks Dr. Alfred Sommer, dean of the Johns Hopkins School of Public Health. And what about Ebola?

If someone could quantify the threat of a smallpox attack, this debate would be winnable. We could weigh the vaccine's hazards against those of an outbreak, and declare one set of hazards more serious. Without that intelligence, it would be hard to justify a peacetime vaccination drive. But nobody is planning one. The new HHS plan recognizes the need for a well-immunized emergency-response network, but it doesn't propose a return to compulsory childhood smallpox shots. It simply envisions letting people choose their own risks. "We'd set it up on a voluntary basis," says Thompson, "and if you wanted it you could have it." Would the risk be worth taking? Maybe not. But as Bicknell points out, most of us face higher risks every day without thinking twice.

It would be nice, of course, if we could have the immunity without the risk. That may soon be possible. The government is stocking up on vaccinia immune globulin, a medicine that can ease adverse reactions to the smallpox vaccines, and funding research to develop entirely new ways of immunizing people. The most promising of the third-generation vaccines—based on a weakened vaccinia strain known as MVA (Modified Vaccinia Ankara)—is already being used in gene therapy and AIDS-vaccine experiments, and even extremely ill patients seem to tolerate it well. After reconfirming MVA's safety, says Fauci, researchers will begin testing its efficacy against smallpox. At the least, he says, it may provide a good booster for people vaccinated decades earlier. When scientists devise a vaccine that is as safe as MVA and as effective as Dryvax, perhaps we'll all take the shot and stop worrying about how to vaccinate the population in 10 days flat. Short of that, no plan can keep us completely immune from danger.

GLOSSARY

anthrax: A disease caused by bacteria, that usually strikes animals such as cattle and sheep but can infect humans and cause death; it is thought to be a likely choice for use in a bioterrorist attack.

antibodies: Substances produced by certain cells in the immune system that help the body identify and destroy invaders such as bacteria and viruses; possession of antibodies to a particular microorganism show that a person has been exposed to that organism, either naturally or in a vaccine.

arbovirus: Short for *arthropod-borne virus*, meaning a disease-causing virus transmitted by mosquitoes, ticks, or similar creatures.

AZT: The abbreviation for *azidothymidine* or *zidovudine*, the first drug developed as a specific treatment for AIDS.

bubonic plague: A disease caused by bacteria; it caused widespread epidemics and pandemics in Europe and Asia, especially from the Middle Ages through the eighteenth century; it is thought to have killed 56 million people in Europe alone.

Centers for Disease Control and Prevention (CDC): The chief U.S. government agency that deals with epidemics, both in the United States and worldwide; its headquarters are in Atlanta, Georgia.

cholera: An epidemic disease caused by bacteria that produces diarrhea, vomiting, rapid dehydration, and death if not treated; it is spread by water contaminated with excrement from people with the disease.

dengue: An infectious disease transmitted by mosquitoes that is marked by fever, pains in the joints, and a rash.

diagnosis: The act or procedure of determining the nature of an illness or medical problem.

DNA fingerprinting: The identification of unique sequences of bases in samples of DNA (deoxyribonucleic acid), or genetic material, from an organism, leading to identification of the organism.

Ebola (or Ebola fever): A usually fatal hemorrhagic fever caused by a virus.

encephalitis: An inflammation of the brain, often caused by microorganisms.

endemic disease: An infectious disease that is constantly present in a particular area but does not strike large numbers of people at once.

enzyme: A member of a large group of different proteins from living things that speed up chemical reactions or allow them to take place.

epidemic: An event in which an infectious disease spreads rapidly and strikes many members of a population at once.

epidemiologist: A scientist who studies factors that affect the occurrence of particular diseases in a population or who studies and tracks epidemics.

eradicate: To wipe out completely.

hemorrhagic fever: One of a group of frequently fatal, virus-caused diseases that causes extensive internal bleeding.

HIV: Human immunodeficiency virus, the virus that most scientists hold to be the cause of AIDS.

immune: Able to resist the attack of a particular type of disease-causing microorganism or other parasite.

immune system: The body's defense system against infectious disease and invasion of foreign substances, consisting of cells and chemicals mostly in the blood.

immunity: Resistance to disease or to a particular kind of disease.

incubation period: The period between the time an organism is infected with disease-causing microorganisms and the time the organism shows clear signs of disease; the organism may be able to spread the disease during this period.

infection: The act of invasion by disease-causing microorganisms or other parasites; an illness or medical condition caused by such parasites.

infectious disease: An illness caused by microorganisms or other parasites.

inoculate: To inject a vaccine or serum into the body in order to produce immunity.

malaria: A blood disease caused by a protozoan (protist) parasite and spread by mosquitoes; it causes recurrent fever, weakness, and sometimes death.

microbe: A microorganism, especially one that can cause disease.

molecular biology: The scientific study of the chemical and physical composition, properties, and activities of molecules in living cells.

National Institutes of Health (NIH): A group of large research institutions in Bethesda, Maryland, sponsored by the U.S. government.

outbreak: A sudden occurrence or small epidemic of infectious disease.

pandemic: An epidemic of infectious disease that affects large areas of the world at once.

pathogen: A microorganism or other parasite that can cause disease.

prion: A misshaped protein that many scientists believe can cause brain-destroying illnesses in humans and animals.

pustule: A small swelling on the skin that contains pus, a sign of infection by disease-causing microorganisms.

quarantine: The act of isolating people or animals that have (or are thought to have) an infectious disease in order to keep the disease from spreading.

reservoir: A species of living thing in which a type of disease-causing microorganism can live, without making that species sick, and from which the microorganisms sometimes move out to make other species sick.

salmonella: A group of microorganism species that cause severe diseases of the digestive tract and are usually spread through contaminated food.

smallpox: A frequently fatal infectious disease caused by a virus. Smallpox has produced devastating epidemics throughout history; natural smallpox was eradicated in the late 1970s, but some experts fear that bioterrorists may reintroduce the disease.

strain: A particular subspecies of living things, such as a microorganism.

streptococcus: A type of microorganism that causes sore throats and a variety of other infections.

surveillance: Close watch kept over a person, place, or situation to detect disease.

symptom: A sign of an illness or medical problem, such as fever.

syndrome: A group of symptoms that occur together and may indicate a particular disease.

toxin: A poisonous substance produced by a living thing, such as a disease-causing microorganism.

tuberculosis (TB): A disease caused by bacteria that, in humans, chiefly affects the lungs and is often fatal.

typhus: An infectious disease caused by microorganisms and spread by lice and fleas, producing fever, a rash, headaches, and often death.

vaccine: A mixture containing dead or weakened disease-causing microorganisms, given to a person or animal for the purpose of helping the immune system develop resistance to the type of microorganism present in the vaccine.

vaccinia: A virus, related to the virus that causes smallpox, that produces a mild illness in cows called cowpox; inoculation or vaccination with this virus was used to produce immunity to smallpox.

variola: Smallpox, or the virus that causes smallpox.

vector: An animal, usually an insect, that spreads a particular type of disease-causing microorganism from infected to uninfected living things.

virulence: The degree to which a microorganism is infectious or able to cause severe disease.

virulent: Highly infectious or able to cause severe disease.

World Health Organization (WHO): An agency founded by the United Nations in 1948 for the purpose of advising countries about health care matters; one of its jobs is tracking and attempting to control epidemics of infectious disease throughout the world.

yellow fever: A frequently fatal disease caused by a virus and spread by mosquitoes, producing fever, yellowish (jaundiced) skin, and often death.

zoonoses: Infectious diseases that spread from animals to humans.

zymotics: Infectious diseases that occur in and spread easily through crowds or groups of people who live very close together.

Books

Ronald Bayer and Gerald M. Oppenheimer, *AIDS Doctors: Voices from the Epidemic*. New York: Oxford University Press, 2000.

Steve Connor and Sharon Kingman, *The Search for the Virus*. New York: Viking Penguin, 1989.

Rob DeSalle, ed., *Epidemic! The World of Infectious Disease*. New York: New Press, 1999.

William Dudley and Mary E. Williams, eds, *Opposing Viewpoints: Epidemics*. San Diego: Greenhaven, 1999.

Elizabeth W. Etheridge, *Sentinel for Health: A History of the Centers for Disease Control*. Berkeley and Los Angeles: University of California Press, 1992.

Paul W. Ewald, *Evolution of Infectious Disease*. New York: Oxford University Press, 1994.

Douglas A. Feldman and Julia Wang Miller, *The AIDS Crisis: A Documentary History*. Westport, CT: Greenwood, 1998.

Laurie Garrett, *The Coming Plague: Newly Emerging Diseases in a World Out of Balance*. New York: Penguin Books, 1994.

Lynette Iezzoni, *Influenza 1918: The Worst Epidemic in American History*. New York: TV Books, 1999.

Arno Karlen, *Man and Microbes: Disease and Plagues in History and Modern Times*. New York: Jeremy P. Tarcher/Putnam, 1995.

Joseph P. McCormick and Susan Fisher-Hoch, *Level 4: Virus Hunters of the CDC*. Atlanta: Turner, 1996.

William H. McNeill, *Plagues and Peoples*. New York: Anchor/ Doubleday, 1998.

Andrew Nikiforuk, *The Fourth Horseman: A Short History of Epidemics, Plagues, and Other Scourges*. London: Phoenix/Orion, 1993.

Michael B.A. Oldstone, *Viruses, Plagues, and History*. New York: Oxford University Press, 1998.

David Perlin and Ann Cohen, *The Complete Idiot's Guide to Dangerous Diseases and Epidemics*. Upper Saddle River, NJ: Alpha Books/Pearson Education, 2002.

C.J. Peters and Mark Olshaker, *Virus Hunter: Thirty Years of Battling Hot Viruses Around the World*. New York: Anchor Books/Bantam Doubleday Dell, 1997.

Richard Preston, *The Hot Zone*. New York: Random House, 1994.

Frank Ryan, *Virus X: Tracking the New Killer Plagues*. Boston: Little, Brown, 1997.

Susan Scott and Christopher J. Duncan, *Biology of Plagues: Evidence from Historical Populations*. New York: Cambridge University Press, 2001.

Paul D. Stolley and Tamar Laskey, *Investigating Disease Patterns: The Science of Epidemiology*. New York: Scientific American Library, 1998.

Sheldon Watts, *Epidemics and History: Disease, Power, and Imperialism*. New Haven, CT: Yale University Press, 1998.

Christopher Wills, *Yellow Fever, Black Goddess: The Coevolution of People and Plagues*. Reading, MA: Helix Books/Addison-Wesley, 1996.

Charles-Edward Amory Winslow, *The Conquest of Epidemic Disease: A Chapter in the History of Ideas*. Madison: University of Wisconsin Press, 1980.

Diane Yancey, *The Hunt for Hidden Killers: Ten Cases of Medical Mystery*. Brookfield, CT: Millbrook, 1994.

Lisa Yount, ed., *Discovery of the AIDS Virus*. San Diego: Greenhaven, 2002.

Periodicals

George J. Armelagos, "The Viral Superhighway," *Sciences*, January/February 1998.

Shannon Brownlee, "The Disease Busters," *U.S. News & World Report*, March 27, 1995.

Geoff Butcher, "'Million Murdering Death': How Malaria Has Impacted Mankind's Progress," *History Today*, April 1998.

John Carey, "Ready for the Next Bug?" *Business Week*, September 16, 2002.

Centers for Disease Control and Prevention, "Protecting the Nation's Health in an Era of Globalization: CDC's Global Infectious Disease Strategy: Executive Summary," 2002. Available online at www.cdc.gov.

Rachel Cohen, "An Epidemic of Neglect," *Multinational Monitor*, June 2002.

Jared Diamond, "The Arrow of Disease," *Discover*, October 1992.

Andrew P. Dobson and E. Robin Carper, "Infectious Diseases and Human Population History," *BioScience*, February 1996.

Catherine Dold, "The Cholera Lesson," *Discover*, February 1999.

Patricia Gadsby, "Fear of Flu," *Discover*, January 1999.

Geoffrey P. Garnett and Edward C. Holmes, "The Ecology of Emergent Infectious Disease," *BioScience*, February 1996.

Denise Grady, "Death at the Corners," *Discover*, December 1993.

Thomas J. Johnson, "From Scythian Poisoned Arrows to Anthrax Dispersal Bombs, Biological Warfare Has Always Been with Us," *Military History*, August 2002.

Erik Larson, "The Flu Hunters," *Time*, February 23, 1998.

Eugene Linden, "Global Fever," *Time*, July 8, 1996.

Robert Matthews, "Millennium Bugs with a Deadly Bite," *UNESCO Courier*, September 1999.

Charles L. Mee Jr., "How a Mysterious Disease Laid Low Europe's Masses," *Smithsonian*, February 1990.

Francois-Xavier Meslin, Klaus Stohr, and P. Formenty, "Emerging Zoonoses," *World Health*, January/February 1997.

Wendy Orent, "Escape from Moscow," *Sciences*, May/June 1998.

———, "The Return of Smallpox," *American Prospect*, December 3, 2001.

Tara O'Toole, Michael Mair, and Thomas V. Inglesby, "Shining Light on 'Dark Winter,'" *Clinical Infectious Diseases*, April 1, 2002.

David Pimentel et al., "Ecology of Increasing Disease," *BioScience*, October 1998.

Peter Radetsky, "Last Days of the Wonder Drugs," *Discover*, November 1998.

Leslie Roberts, "The Comeback Plague," *U.S. News & World Report*, March 27, 2000.

Ellen Ruppel Shell, "Resurgence of a Deadly Disease," *Atlantic Monthly*, August 1997.

Gunjan Sinha and Burkhard Bilger, "Skeletons from the Attic," *Sciences*, September/October 1996.

Gary Taubes, "Apocalypse Not," *Science*, November 7, 1997.

———, "Malarial Dreams," *Discover*, March 1998.

Time International, "Stalking a Killer," September 30, 2002.

John Travis, "Spying Diseases from the Sky," *Science News*, August 2, 1997.

Mark Wheelis, "Biological Warfare at the 1346 Siege of Caffa," *Emerging Infectious Diseases*, September 2002.

Websites

Centers for Disease Control and Prevention, www.bt.cdc.gov. This website includes information about natural infectious diseases, biological weapons, and how to protect oneself against attack.

International Society for Infectious Diseases, www.promedmail. org. The society's website offers data on recent outbreaks of infectious diseases such as West Nile fever, Ebola, and anthrax in different parts of the world.

Outbreak, www.outbreak.org. Outbreak's website provides information and links to sites related to infectious diseases.

World Health Organization, www.who.int. The World Health Organization is the official public source for news of infectious disease outbreaks around the world.

INDEX

AIDS. *See* HIV/AIDS
anthrax, 78
Archidamus, 43
arthropod-borne infections, 22–23
   WHO surveillance for, 92
Athens, Plague of, 13, 24, 43–48
Aztecs, 13

Bicknell, Bill, 107
Biggs, Herman, 59
Black Death, 29
   map of spread of, 14
Brushingham, J.P., 59
bubonic plague, 29
   in London, 49–53
   spread of, in Europe, 14
Bush administration
   smallpox vaccination program
      of, 102–103

Callisher, Charlie, 89, 90, 91
Carlsson, Mark, 106
case control studies, 38–39
Centers for Disease Control and
   Prevention (CDC), 35
Chileshe, Simon, 68
Chiluba, Frederick, 71
cholera
   annual deaths from, 30
   return of, in Latin America,
      33–34, 96
cities
   evolution of epidemics and,
      18–21, 26–27

climate change
   impact of, on infectious diseases,
      33–34
Cohen, Ann, 77
Coming Plague, The (Garrett), 31
*Complete Idiot's Guide to Dangerous
   Diseases and Epidemics, The* (Perlin
   and Cohen), 77
computers
   in disease surveillance, 79–80
   in epidemic tracking, 40
Copeland, Royal, 59
Cortés, Hernán, 13
Cowley, Geoffrey, 101
Cragg, Georgina, 55
Cuba
   dengue epidemic in, 91

diseases
   communicable
      identification of new forms of,
         32, 78–79
      sources of information on,
         97–98
   crowd, 19, 21
   sexually transmitted, 21
   spread of, 13–14, 24–25, 28–29
   see also specific diseases
DNA technology. *See* genetic
   technology

Ebola fever, 15, 61–65
   in Gabon, 89
El Niño, 33